HOMESTEADING

A Resource Guide to Homesteading Opportunities
in the United States

(As Small Scale, Homestead and Urban Farming)

Lillian Porterfield

Published by Harry Barnes

Lillian Porterfield

All Rights Reserved

Homesteading: A Resource Guide to Homesteading Opportunities in the United States (As Small Scale, Homestead and Urban Farming)

ISBN 978-1-7778032-6-1

All rights reserved. No part of this guide may be reproduced in any form without permission in writing from the publisher except in the case of brief quotations embodied in critical articles or reviews.

Legal & Disclaimer

The information contained in this book is not designed to replace or take the place of any form of medicine or professional medical advice. The information in this book has been provided for educational and entertainment purposes only.

The information contained in this book has been compiled from sources deemed reliable, and it is accurate to the best of the Author's knowledge; however, the Author cannot guarantee its accuracy and validity and cannot be held liable for any errors or omissions. Changes are periodically made to this book. You must consult your doctor or get professional medical advice before using any of the suggested remedies, techniques, or information in this book.

Upon using the information contained in this book, you agree to hold harmless the Author from and against any damages, costs, and expenses, including any legal fees potentially resulting from the application of any of the information provided by this guide. This disclaimer applies to any damages or injury caused by the use and application, whether directly or indirectly, of any advice or information presented, whether for breach of contract, tort, negligence, personal injury, criminal intent, or under any other cause of action.

You agree to accept all risks of using the information presented inside this book. You need to consult a professional medical practitioner in order to ensure you are both able and healthy enough to participate in this program.

Table of Contents

INTRODUCTION 1

CHAPTER 1: WHAT IS HOMESTEADING 2

CHAPTER 2: HOMESTEAD OR HOMESTEADING 23

CHAPTER 3: THE BENEFITS OF BACKYARD HOMESTEADING 35

CHAPTER 4: BACKYARD LIVESTOCK FOR FOOD 44

CHAPTER 5: EFFICIENT SPACE 53

CHAPTER 6: POULTRY AND LIVESTOCK 59

CHAPTER 7: PRESERVING YOUR HARVEST 63

CHAPTER 8: PLAN FOR MAKING YOUR OWN BACKYARD FARM 85

CHAPTER 9: TYPES OF HOMESTEAD GARDENING 92

CHAPTER 10: GARDENING TIPS AND STRATEGY TO MAXIMIZE YOUR HOMESTEAD HARVEST 118

CHAPTER 11: 10 EASY WAYS TO GROW PLANTS FOR THE BEGINNING EDIBLE LANDSCAPE GARDENER 137

CHAPTER 12: RAISING CHICKEN 144

CHAPTER 13: STARTING TO HOMESTEAD 171

CONCLUSION 180

Introduction

Homesteading for beginners, For those in the environmentally aware circles, there is a term that is making a comeback of sorts albeit in a slightly different meaning than was originally intended.

That term is homesteading.

Homesteading was originally a US government legislation that gave away free land to people who took large tracts of rural land and then converted it into their primary landholding and place of residence.

It was a huge success as it helped develop some of the largely rural parts of the country years ago.

Chapter 1: What Is Homesteading

Homesteading is more of a continuum. The broadest concept, after all, is that it is a lifestyle with a dedication to self-sufficiency. It may include growing and storing food; using the sun, wind or water for your electricity; and even producing your fabric and clothes. Some homestays never want to use money; they want to make or barter for anything they need. Some may take a more cautious approach, and while striving to support themselves with as best as they can, they may be comfortable having some resources and working for pay — either as an end target or during the transition to homesteading.

Urban and suburban homesteading is a type of homesteading; people living in the city or suburbs may often find themselves homesteaders, and seek to cater for their own needs within the limits of a small residential house and yard or even a small town estate.

Homesteaders don't inherently all have the same homesteading beliefs and motivations and can be a mixed group. Some may be retiring from a lucrative career that enables them to have the money to invest in the infrastructure needed to support themselves fully on the land. Many can come home with little, building a scrappy refuge to provide for themselves in the face of economic hardship. These two situations might look very different, yet both are considered homesteaders.

History Of Homesteading

Land-grant legislation similar to the Homestead Acts had been introduced by Northern Republicans before the Civil War but had been thwarted repeatedly by Southern Democrats in Congress who required Western lands available to slave-owners to purchase. The Homestead Act of 1860 passed in Congress but President James Buchanan, a Republican, vetoed it. The bill passed and was signed into law by President Abraham Lincoln (May 20, 1862) after the Southern states seceded from the Union in 1861 (and their members had left Congress). The first person to lodge a lawsuit under the new act was Daniel Freeman.

The federal government granted 1,6 million homes between 1862 and 1934 and allocated 270,000,000 acres (420,000 sq mi) of public land for private possession. That was a minimum of 10 per cent of all U.S. property. Except in Alaska, where it continued until 1986, Homesteading was abandoned in 1976. Around 40 per cent of the applicants who began the process was able to complete it and gain rights to their homesteaded property after paying a small fee in cash.

The "yeoman farmer" principle of Jeffersonian democracy was already a strong force in American politics in the 1840-1850s, with many politicians hoping that a homestead act would help to raise the amount of "virtuous yeomen." The Free Soil Movement of 1848–52 and the emerging Republican Party after 1854 insisted that the new lands opening up in the west be made available to individual farmers, rather than rich planters who would grow them through the help of slavery driving the yeomen farmers into marginal lands.

Southern Democrats had constantly resisted (and defeated) previous attempts for a homestead law because they feared they would be free. It was signed by Abraham Lincoln on May 20, 1862, when the most vocal opposition in Congress, the southern states, had been eliminated following the Secession of the United States. His main supporters were Andrew Johnson, George Henry Evans and Horace Greeley. The popular term "Give Yourself a Farm" was invented by George Henry Evans to attract campaign support.

The homestead was a field of federal property in the West (usually 160 acres or 65 ha) given to any resident of the United States who desired to settle and cultivate the property. The statute (and those that follow) involved a three-step procedure: apply, update the land and file a patent (deed). Any person who had never taken up arms against the U.S. government (including freed slaves since the fourteenth amendment) and was at least 21 years of age, or the head of a household, may qualify for a federal land grant. Females were free. Over five years, the tenant had to live on the property and provide proof of changes made. In 7 years the cycle needed to be complete.

The act stripped the Native Americans of most of their land and natural wealth in the United States as a result of its redistribution and selling to mainly white settlers

Benefits of homesteading

Homesteading has a range of legal and financial advantages, including the ability to improve your quality of life including satisfaction.

1. Homestead Exemptions Homesteaders can make use of something called an exception for homesteads in some US states. This allows homeowners to hedge from creditors and taxes the value of their home and property.

This profit always carries on to a partner if the householder dies. Homestead advantages are for your and your spouse's life, as long as you continue to own the house.

That means homesteading could theoretically give you something called protection from forced selling. That ensures that whether you default on a loan or other obligation, creditors can't compel you to sell your house to pay your debts.

That does typically not shield you from different forms of loans, such as defaulted property taxes or foreclosure on mortgages.

Some states allow you to exempt all of your property from property taxes. For other instances, you're protected up to a reasonable sum, like the first $50,000 to $75,000 of the appraised value of your house.

Given that exemptions from homesteads vary too widely from state to state, you can consult a lawyer or accountant before making any financial decisions relating to your property.

2. Safety Getting the right to your property and house provides a better sense of protection for certain homestays.

With reduced expenses and taxes, and the freedom to be self-sufficient and live off the farm, homesteading will give you a sense of stability.

By living the lifestyle of homesteading, you would, of course, have lower bills.

Homesteaders continue to have smaller wages but they do not even have to work a traditional job because they have significantly lower expenses.

3. Homesteaders congratulate themselves on finding a piece of land to call their own. Most couldn't picture renting a little apartment, wanting to get their land where they could take care of their lives.

4. Less stress Like most people living in the region, homesteaders describe experiencing far less stress than those living in noisy, busy cities and urban centres.

Imagine the sounds of birds chirping and cattle circling your house, instead of heavy cars and police sirens.

5. More Environmentally Aware Homesteaders are more closely linked to nature than those living in the area. They know where their food comes from because they always produce much of it on their own.

As a result, they have an opportunity to take better care of the environment and to make sure that their agricultural activities are safe.

This means they will continue to support their land for the rest of their lives, and hopefully also their children's lives.

6. Good Physical Health Running a house needs much more physical work than a job in the workplace or more employees in the community in that case.

Combine this with the fact this homeowners usually consume balanced organic meals they make themselves and have much less ability to indulge in packaged foods such as pizza or chips.

Less tension, daily physical fitness and a balanced diet are all key factors in staying well fit into old age, and enjoying a long life.

7. Improved self-confidence Building a homestead would take a whole range of new skills and interests you've never had before.

Such new skills will allow you to become more able and self-sufficient. And as a result, your self-esteem and self-confidence will undoubtedly grow significantly.

It's not easy to home settle. There's a steep learning curve to learn all the new skills you'll need. At first, it can be intimidating and maybe even frustrating. But all of these struggles will help you develop into a stronger human being.

To know that you are self-sufficient and completely in charge of your fate is a very rewarding feeling.

For certain homesteaders, civilization and the power grid could vanish tomorrow, and they will still live the same lifestyle exactly.

8. The Bonding Homesteading family will get the family back together. Imagine no longer wanting to go to work at a workplace all day.

Instead, alongside your spouse and children, you can spend your day doing chores and taking care of your house.

That means a lot of chances for each other to talk and enjoy quality time.

Homesteading does not build the ideal household, automatically. When you choose your room, you are also likely to have disagreements and time.

But after it's all said and done, a family who spends time together during the day and sits down to share a meal is likely to feel closer to each other because of it.

Disadvantages of homesteading

We're going to continue the negatives with something that might not be that bad, but in certain people's opinion, it may be a downside; the smell. If you live in a rural area and want to buy your animals, you will end up with the scent that goes with them. The lovely scent of manure in your home can fill your days and some people can't handle this. There are air diffusers and other items that you can purchase to try to block these smells, as you can see on www.aromatech.com.

However, if you have a sensitive nose it can take a while to get used to and feel fairly off-putting.

Another big downside to living in a homestead is that you're completely cut off from modern society. This ensures that you do not have access to a host of items that you're used to having close by. Rural life means you don't have access to shops and quick treatment. Still, there's the entire conundrum of internet and phone as well. It's difficult to get broadband delivered in remote areas, which means you might pay for internet that's bad, losing a lot of time.

Finally, living in a homestead requires a lot of hard work and commitment. If you want to devote yourself completely to this way of life then your days will be filled with physical activities requiring tons of resources. It is not as laid back as you would have thought! It requires careful preparation and an understanding of how to stop overwhelming.

Knowing the pros and cons of living in a household will help you make the best decision when it comes to homesteading.

At the end of the day, some people suit this way of life better than others. If you don't have any connections to the city and want to stay away from it all and start being more self-sufficient, then it's fine. But, if you rely heavily on digital technologies, the internet, and getting connected to it all – then it's not perfect for you!

Reasons to Homestead

• You see the potential destruction of the coming modern society and hope that even if modern luxury goods and systems collapse, you should be prepared to live as "normally" as possible.

• To reduce the amount of electricity required and use solar, wind, or hydropower to reduce or even eliminate dependence on the grid that may collapse at any time.

• Be good at growing and/or improving your food to ensure that after the grocery store shelves are empty or food rations are implemented, you and your family will have a food source.

• Reduced dependence on the government, which appears to be acting in ways that are increasingly not in the best interests of its citizens.

• Avoid high food prices and/or high utility costs.

• Avoid the impact of genetically modified organisms on food, and more organic diet

• To escape the false American dream of work, you hate to have a property that has little time to own (large house, limousine, swimming pool, camper, etc.).

In some ways, we are lucky that modern house fixing is not all or all the adventures of those early house fixers. At least not yet. Those who wish to become housewives today can do it in stages and can choose how far away from the dependents we want to be. For most people, choosing to be self-reliant or disconnected from the grid does not mean getting rid of the shackles of modern society, but more of being able to live "normally" when needed.

Reasons Not To Homestead

I'm not going to lie and tell you it's just rainbows and butterflies. Heck, little house on the prairie had a heartbreak share of it. Here are the two reasons I'd advise anyone away from home:

IT'S HARD WORK, the weather is not waiting for you, the babies are not waiting for you. You work 10 to 12 hours a day, putting up fruit if it's canning season. When it's down, you're chopping down firewood before you allow your weapons to go. That is a lot of hard, manual labour. And while this labour may be healthy for you, the days you want to leave will be coming.

IT'S HARD Not just physically hard but it's mentally hard. It is never easy to lose one animal. It's never easy to see one sick animal. You're going to waste endless hours and money growing a garden, only to have squash beetles mow it down. You're trying to raise a flock of 2-day-old hens – placing 6 months of caring, treatment, and food in them before they can begin laying – to get them wiped out by a predator.

The storm floods. The heat is just going to scorch. Animals are expected to die. That's going to disrupt everything. You're going to get sick or wounded and watch something collapse. So the following day, you are going to wake up and try again. Why? For what?

Tips On Homesteading

Are you new to building your homestead, or are you talking about building your own? Know from others, and stop making repetitive mistakes. Check out some of the best advice from experienced homesteaders for those considering beginning a self-sufficient homestead.

Many people who get discouraged and exhausted by homesteading take on more than they can do adequately, then feel stressed and stretched too thin. Set your eyes on a few pretty good targets each season, instead of distributing your resources through several targets. You could end up broken and fractured.

Try using a book called "The Weekend Homesteader" to handle tasks one weekend at a time rather than biting out more than you can chew. Several subjects include: • Setting goals for your small farm and household • Setting livestock to raise • Designing your farm is perfect for you?

Are you cut out for being a homesteader? Consider long and hard before you start on what is a love-work. Be willing to go through long, hard hours of manual labour, always frustrating and unpleasant, for the pure pleasure of being able to fulfil your own needs. If like most of us do, you've grown up in a western culture, that can be a big transition and not one that other people can quickly achieve.

Plan for any income While you may initially fantasize that you will supply you and your family with anything you need and never pay a dime, that's not true. You'll have to realize that you'll have expenses that will need capital, particularly when you move to a self-sustaining homestead.

Consider the way you enjoy living, too. Will you want to go to the restaurants or go out to dance? Will you love travelling or watching cultural events? You'll need some money to afford life-long stuff you can't barter or make yourself.

Eschew Debt Borrowing money goes against any idea on which the aim of self-sufficiency is based. Typically speaking, people who wish to be homestead tend to be able to disengage from the financial system and work as little as possible for income. Instead of using currency, farmers grow their crops, and maybe barter for things like clothing and other products that are needed.

Keep The Expenses Minimal This is relevant when contemplating the properties you own (most people who want to purchase their land or house). Will you purchase land with cash and even build a house with cash on it yourself? Or are you going to purchase a house that is already constructed on some acreage? If you are considering buying your homestead property on a mortgage, how are you going to cover the mortgage? Will you pay it off in a shorter period than 30 years?

Remember how your house will be heated and cooled, and how it will provide electricity. The use of renewable sources of energy such as sun, wind, or geothermal will substantially reduce the expenses. Many homesteaders refuse to be "on the grid," as a vital aspect of their self-sufficiency ambitions, preferring to supply their electricity. You will need to spend some time on your homestead determining whether you will be caring for these needs.

Embrace Simplicity and Give Up on Aesthetics. You have one goal, as a homesteader: self-sufficiency. The hours you spend keeping things beautiful are hours you should be doing practical stuff to achieve your self-sufficiency target.

If you place pressure on yourself to make your household look like it belongs in "Great Homesteads and Gardens," when doing all the required tasks in a day to manage a household, that's an impossible task. If you don't excel you are likely to get discouraged and exhausted. Let go of the lingering commitment to items that look neat and coexistent. It'll help you obtain more.

Around the same time, if you're chugging along, making good strides towards the overall target of self-sufficiency, not exhausted, and being able to keep stuff tidy and safe to boot, then perfect. The point is not to fret about it.

For a homesteader, a life of comfort and glamour is not in the cards. Homesteading is all about the belief that you are not helped by exchanging time for money, as well as using your resources to provide specifically for your needs. Simple life, or life simply on earth, involves growing one's belongings and costs and learning to be content with only satisfying your needs, and letting go of wants and consumption.

Time Worked Means Self-Sufficiency If you hate the hours spent nurturing cattle, canning vegetables, and cutting wood — then it's not for you to be homesteading. Alternatively, imagine the end aim to be a hobby farm where your aim is merely to appreciate the farming pieces you don't hate, without self-sufficiency. Or perhaps a small farm is the right choice, where you focus on both earning money and farming.

Separate time in your mind from money. Sure, you would have worked for maybe $15 an hour, but then, by raising your chickens, you only worked the equivalent of $5 an hour. The entire argument is that you have lived on your terms with yourself and you are building something that goes deeper than exchanging your time for an hourly wage.

Roll Comedy With the Punches is sweet. Laugh, every day. Do not go into homesteading on a big horse and feeling that you are equal to everyone else. When things go bad with the chickens pooping all over the front steps and the foxes start targeting your hens, try to maintain calm.

You'll need to take it easy on yourself and be fine if you don't meet your goals as soon as you think. Sit down and restructure your plan to reflect new goals and new timelines when needed. All are flexible. Enjoy the process of getting a little bit of self-sufficiency at a time.

Chapter 2: Homestead Or Homesteading

There are many definitions and ideas of what a homestead is. In a historical context, a "homestead" was defined as a parcel of land (typically 160 acres) that was granted to any US citizen willing to move West to settle on and farm the land for at least five years, as part of the Homestead Act of 1862.

In more modern terms, the act of homesteading is used to describe an agrarian and largely self-sufficient lifestyle. Homesteading activities typically include growing and preserving food crops, cooking meals from scratch, raising animals, making homemade medicines, personal care products, perhaps even clothing, and an overall goal to "live off the land". Homesteaders may also barter and trade for the things they cannot produce themselves.

Homesteaders come in many forms and styles these days. Some homesteaders have acres of land to play with (and maintain), while urban homesteaders are challenged and creative in smaller spaces. There are some hard-core, very traditional homesteaders that attempt to live a fully self-sufficient, zero-waste, off-grid, or near "prepper" status life. Then there are your hobby homesteaders, who are simply drawn to this lifestyle and enjoy it as a light-hearted escape from their usual 9-5 "real life". All versions of homesteading are awesome and acceptable! I'd say we are somewhere in between.

A homestead can mean different things to different people. But in a broad sense, homesteading is about living a self-sufficient lifestyle. For most people, the main aspects of a homestead are owning their land and the buildings on it, and doing small-scale farming with the goal of being self-sufficient, or at least limiting their reliance on outside sources.

Although homesteading typically applies to farms, it's also possible to be an urban homesteader by practicing sustainable living techniques, urban agriculture, and a frugal lifestyle.

Some people believe that homesteading is more defined by the lifestyle choices that you make, rather than whether you live in the country or the city. In the UK, what's called homesteading is often referred to as smallholding. Or less frequently as crofting.

Homesteaders practice subsistence agriculture and often preserve their own food that they harvest to last them through the winter.So skills like canning and pickling are essential for homesteaders to have.

They may even produce their own clothing, textiles, and other crafts. Either to use within their own home or to sell to generate a little bit of extra income.

Homesteading is differentiated from living in a commune or village because of its isolation, both geographically and socially. A homestead typically only houses a single family, or at most, their extended family.Whereas a commune usually has a group of people living together who share responsibilities and possessions but are only loosely connected.

Homesteaders tend to live a more independent life, and may only venture into town once a week or less for supplies or to see friends. This is particularly true for homesteaders who choose not to have a job and get all the income needed to pay for taxes and other expenses from work done on their own land.

Homesteads are far more likely to rely on renewable energy sources like wind or solar electricity than the average home. In addition to growing their own vegetables and livestock, the idea of being completely "off-grid" is a massive appeal to a lot of homesteaders.

STEPS TO START A HOMESTEAD

EVALUATE YOUR PROPERTY

Every property will come with its unique strengths and challenges. When you first set out to start a homestead – what type of property are you working with? Do you already own land, or are you still on the hunt to find a slice of Earth to call your own? Are you currently in your forever home, or do you hope to move again someday soon?

TEMPORARY VS FOREVER

While you will not want to invest a huge amount of money or energy into a rental or temporary space, don't let it stop you from practicing at least some homesteading activities. For example, when we lived in rental accommodations, we still built a couple of raised garden beds. We also grew food in containers, and started composting. This small introduction enabled us to learn some basics of gardening before buying our first home. Just be sure to check with your landlord before doing anything too permanent.

We know this current property isn't our forever home, but we certainly haven't let that stop us from enjoying it to the fullest while we are here! Before we were able to have an extensive garden, we stocked up on seasonal produce at local farmers markets to practice various food preservation techniques. You can also learn to sew, craft, brew kombucha, or make homemade sourdough no matter your living situation.

A four part image collage showing what one can do in a rental property with limited space. The images vary from getting the necessary supplies to build raised beds such as wood and soil, filling the raised bed with soil once it is built, planting out the raised beds with various plants of choice, in this case it was tomatoes, squash, peppers,and basil, and finally using containers to grow vegetables. They can easily be moved and don't take up as much space.

SIZE, RESTRICTIONS, & LAYOUT

Now, think about the property size.A modestly-sized property will be more manageable in regards to maintenance, but may also limit the activities you can do on it such as what types of animals you can raise. Goats, cows, or pigs would not be happy in our 1/5 acre town lot. Nor could we legally keep them. Be sure to familiarize yourself with your town regulations regarding livestock, poultry, bee-keeping, or even things like having a farm stand or collecting rainwater if those are things you're interested in doing.

Now, assuming you do have some property to work with. It's time to make the most of it! Before diving into any permanent projects, be sure to take time to sit back and observe first. For example, you should evaluate an area's sun exposure and source of shade before installing a veggie garden. Also keep in mind how the sun's path will change with the seasons.

Spend time wandering about in your space. How do you want it to eventually look, feel, and function? While nothing needs to be set in stone now, try to dream up your optimal layout – which should be convenient and functional.

A great example of a thoughtful and purposeful layout is through permaculture design, as shown below. You won't want your farm animals directly next to the house. They may be stinky or noisy. Yet you don't want them so far away that it becomes a trek to go visit and care for them, especially if you live in an area with cold winters. Something you will visit frequently, such as a kitchen herb garden, would be ideal just outside the front or back door. Keep your compost area fairly accessible, but not outside your bedroom or kitchen window. I think you get the idea.

MAKE A LIST OF PROJECTS & IDEAS

If you're dreaming to start a homestead, two types of thoughts are likely going through your head. One, you're fantasizing about all of the wonderful, healthy, uber-rewarding things that this new lifestyle will bring you. And it will! I promise. But two You are also fretting over all the skills, tools, money, time, or other resources you may not have to make all of those dreams come true right now. Here is the deal: pretty much no one does. Not right at first, and not all at once.

Remember that creating a homestead is a process, and this is just the start.

Example Homesteading Projects & Goals
- Create a veggie garden space
- Plant an herb garden

- Plant fruit trees or an orchard
- Start a compost area, worm bin, compost tumbler (or all of the above)
- Create a pollinator bed, area, or even a meadow full of flowers
- Learn how to ferment, can, dehydrate and/or pickle your harvests
- Adopt chickens, goats, sheep, rabbits, pigs, cows, or other "farm animals"
- Build a barn, stables, or other auxiliary structures
- Create a root cellar or large pantry
- Learn how to make kombucha, homemade sourdough, apple cider vinegar, homemade seasonings, vegetable (or bone) broth, and other useful staples
- Learn how to make natural medicine like Fire Cider and Elderberry Syrup, or personal care products like calendula oil, soap, lotions.
- Start a beehive
- Learn how to sew, knit, crochet, or use natural dyes
- Turn your property in to a Certified Wildlife Habitat

- Build or install a greenhouse or hoop house

- Set up a rainwater collection system system
- Learn how to make compost tea
- Start a farm stand
- Sell homemade goods locally or online
- Host workshops, classes, or homestays to share your knowledge and skills with others

A hand is holding a National Wildlife Federation Certified Wildlife Habitat plaque in front of a view of the front yard garden. There isn't a lot of open space with many plants for pollinators, raised beds for vegetables, shrubs, and trees spaced throughout the area.

A wonderful long-term goal is to turn your property into an ecosystem of its own. But there are usually many smaller (manageable) projects and steps along the way to get there.

PRIORITIZE

Now take just one or two manageable projects at a time, and forget everything else on the list for a while. It is 100% unrealistic (and 7000% stressful) to try and do everything at once, within a year, or even within a couple of years! That is, unless you are diving in to start a homestead full-time with unlimited resources and help. Where to begin? Well, your priorities are personal. This journey to start a homestead is all about what you want to do, and when you want to do it. There are no rules.

Will this simply be a hobby homestead, or do you intend to make a living from your land? That will obviously influence how seriously or quickly you approach projects, and which ones to focus on first.For example, do you hope to sell eggs locally? Then building a secure chicken coop and establishing a flock will be at the top of your list.

Certain homestead projects will dictate the order or timeline for others. For instance, you shouldn't set up a beehive until you have a healthy pollinator garden, orchard, or other nectar and pollen-producing plants established first.

Circumstance will also drive your priorities. Like: "Oh crap, the irrigation line broke! I guess it is time to brush up on our plumbing skills…" Or that moment when your kitchen counter is overflowing with homegrown tomatoes, but you've never preserved tomatoes before. Evidently, the time to dive in and learn is now.

Chapter 3: The Benefits Of Backyard Homesteading

If you ask any homesteader how homesteading makes them feel, they will likely tell you that they feel blessed. And the truth is you won't know just how fortunate they feel until you become a homesteader yourself. You start reaping the benefits of getting your food directly from your backyard farm. The many benefits of backyard homesteading are enough reasons for you to start backyard homesteading if you are still on the fence. Undoubtedly, making a transition from getting your food from the grocery store to getting it from your backyard farm isn't always easy for homesteading beginners. However, it does get better with time.

And then, there is the whole thing with convincing your family about the new vision and goals you have. Most people find it challenging to convince their families of how beneficial their new lifestyle would be once they get started. In this age, it is effortless to come up with different excuses as to why homesteading may not be the right lifestyle for you. For instance, some people don't want to be homesteaders because they think it'll make people see them as hippies. Others simply don't want the inconvenience that comes with being a backyard homesteader, even though the lifestyle is far from being inconvenient.

"Why start a micro-urban farm when you can just get your food from the grocery store?" Well, I can assure you that sourcing the food you consume by yourself, on your own farm, is much more satisfying and helpful than buying stale food from your local grocery store. The best time to begin working on your backyard homesteading plan is NOW, and you shouldn't let anything deter you. Even if you have to start by taking baby steps. And if you experience setbacks, if people will think you're strange because you have decided to be an urban farmer, know that it always ends up being worth it. So, if you need some extra push to start working towards your goals, here are some benefits of backyard homesteading that should convince your family and even you.

Food Awareness

Unsurprisingly, many people in society are unaware of where food comes from and how it arrives at the dinner table. Children, in particular, don't have the slightest hint or clue of where their favorite meals come from. Homesteading is the key to educating your children and your family about food and where it comes from. A micro-urban farm encourages you to develop an intimate connection with the cycle of food production. This knowledge is something every human, no matter how young or old, should have. It helps you understand and appreciate the seemingly trivial achievement of being able to put food on your table. Something is satisfying about knowing where your food comes from. It helps you understand nature more.

In a way, the homesteading experience is also humbling. Homesteaders are usually quick to understand just how finite life is. As a beginner to urban homesteading, you will make a lot of mistakes. These mistakes can be overwhelming. Your livestock will die. Seemingly healthy crops will also die. Structures may collapse, and your plan may fail more than once. The experience is humbling for many people. If you keep chickens, they will likely be attacked and eaten by predators. But, regardless of the failures and lessons, you are going to continue homesteading if you are really keen on it. If anybody tells you there is a way to practice backyard homesteading without making mistakes at all, you should know that person is playing on your naivety. So, as homesteading is a quite humbling journey for people, it helps build perseverance. Urban homesteading is character building.

With backyard homesteading comes a level of freedom that most people haven't achieved in their lifetime. Due to the self-sufficient lifestyle, many homesteaders tend to become relatively independent, usually more than they have ever been.

Becoming an urban homesteader frees you from the centralized food supply. Most homesteaders don't worry about people complaining about the inflation of dairy products in the market. If you have a cow, why do you have to worry about the rising price of milk? Even if beef becomes more expensive, homesteaders don't worry because they know they have their livestock. The increased level of freedom from price-hike at the market makes your heart giddy and happy. It is enough reason to become an urban homesteader today.

Security

To some extent, homesteading offers security during extreme times. It does not matter whether your issue is a small or significant concern; you can always count on homesteading to provide a level of security in terms of foods and skills. If you know any homesteader, then you probably know that they still have a supply of food on hand because: 1) when you grow your food, there is always extra to preserve and store away. 2) Many homesteaders cannot help keeping mason jars and canning supplies. Although your personal food preservations techniques may need a little polishing when you become a homesteader, the fact is that you will always have enough food supply to last you for months, in the pantry, cupboards, basement, and freezer. Plus, some of the skills you hone from becoming a homesteader can be really helpful in extreme survival scenarios.

Work Ethic

Unsurprisingly, homesteading also helps to sharpen your work ethic. You'll agree that one thing that is currently missing in world culture today is a strong work ethic. Go back to the times of our ancestors, and you will find that children started learning all about providing their own food, milking cows and growing crops from the ages of six and seven. In those times, children already knew how to feed animals and train oxen. Nowadays, though, the environment is entirely different. The truth is that children become capable, and they thrive in any situation that encourages them to partake in worthwhile activities. While you should be grateful that your children don't have to go through such intense labor in this age (thanks to technology and advancement), you can't deny that homesteading can help build up your kids with strong work ethics. It doesn't matter how little they do. If there is anything that can help children build themselves up to develop a strong work ethic, it is the responsibility that accompanies growing food. It teaches them and you so much and it comes with the responsibility of ensuring that everyone can eat and survive; and the livestock you raise depends on you for their own survival, day after day.

Healthy, Tasty Food

Food that comes directly from your own farm tastes better than food from the grocery store. Eggs that come from your own poultry looks a lot healthier and taste better than store-bought eggs, for good reasons. If you know anyone who keeps chickens, then you should know how bright and beautiful the yolk from healthy backyard hens are. The taste is always incomparable. The depth of the difference between homegrown food and conventional food is simply incredible. Homesteading food tastes good. Homesteading also teaches you to be appreciative of what you have. When you understand the level of work that goes into growing your own food – from planting the seeds to caring for the seedlings and nurturing them until they mature – it is hard not to show appreciation and be grateful. Nothing nurtures gratitude and satisfaction more than knowing the amount of hard work that goes into providing your family and loved ones with food to eat. Inadvertently, this also teaches you to treat your crops better and appreciate their values.

There are many more benefits of backyard homesteading, but this should be about enough to convince you and anyone else you would like to convince on the reasons why backyard homesteading is ideal for your family. In the next chapter, we discuss how you can get started with backyard homesteading. What is the first thing you do to start homesteading in your urban home? Let's find out in the subsequent chapter.

Chapter 4: Backyard Livestock For Food

If you are interested in reducing your dependence on the outside world, then you should raise animals because the animals can provide you:

Healthy meat and poultry without any hormones

Fresh milk and eggs to make your morning happy

You can get fresh cheese and butter as by-products

The animals will bring joy to your whole family

You can get mowed down grass and fertilizers for the plants

It is easy to multiply them because their population can be increased easily

Animals that You Can Raise

Following are some animals that you can easily raise in your farmhouse:

Raise Goats

Goats are the excellent choice to rise while living homestead because these require low maintenance and they can take care of themselves. There will be no need to make some extra expenses because goats love to eat bushes, trees, scrub and aromatic herbs. The sheep and cattle may starve to death in the absence of a particular food, but the goats can survive easily. The goat milk is good for the elder people, patients and children having allergies to cow milk. The ulcer patients can also use goat milk. The fat and casein of the goat milk are really easy to digest as compared to the cow milk.

The goats offer lots of benefits, and they will not require anything in return. They can eat your wild plants and offer you milk. You can play with them and use their meat as well. It is quite rewarding to raise urban goats because of convenience in raising them.

There are basically six types of goats, including Nubians, Alpines, Togenburgs, Oberhaslis, LaManchas, and Saanens. If you are looking for the best breed, then you can choose Nubian because these can give quality goat milk. These types of goats can give milk in maximum quantity.

Raising Cows

If you want to raise a cow, think twice about it because it will be your biggest responsibility in the farm. You need to arrange fodder for it and milk it twice a day. The cow dung can be used as compost can be your biggest responsibility. You need to spend more time with the cow because the cow will require your most attention. The cow will be the source of more profit because you can make cheese and butter with the milk of cows. You can sell these items in the market to earn more profit.

Raise Sheep in Your Farmhouse

The sheep are very good to keep because they can support themselves easily. They can live in the grass and become very fat. They will not make any demands from you unless the ground is covered with the snow. These are very cheap to keep and it will be good to have a native breed to the country. You can get meat and fur from sheep to make some profit.

Raise Chickens

You can raise the chicken on the healthy way by providing them enough space to flap their wings and scrap. It will be good to keep dust baths and keep them in a cage. If you want to enjoy eggs for the whole year, feed your chicken with a handful of grains in the evening and give high protein food items in the morning. They will like to eat grass and hatch little chicks. If you want to keep your garden secure, then don't leave chickens in your garden otherwise they will spoil everything.

It will be good to have a cock among your hens and give plenty of space to them in the fields and woods. The hens will constantly produce eggs, but you can also get their meat if needed. The extra supply of eggs can be sold in the market to earn some money.

Raise Geese

It is very easy to raise geese in your farmhouse because it requires low maintenance and easy to keep. The three geese in a pen with one opposite gender will live happily on the grass. You can feed those grains and keep them in your home to avoid foxes. The grain is not necessary fro geese, but you should throw the grains in the night to lure them; otherwise they will be attacked by rats and foxes. The rats can steal the eggs and young geese, but the mother goose may protect their young geese under features. The geese may start laying in the February or March. You can keep any animal or bird in your livestock as per your convenience. You need to think about the available space and maintenance cost before selecting any bird or animal for your livestock.

Homesteaders like to raise livestock to get eggs, milk, meat and other byproducts. These are healthy to use as food and if you have something surplus, you can sell in the market. There are a few simple lessons to raise livestock for food:

Select Your Livestock

There are numerous options from laying hens to chicken, cattle, sheep, rabbits and fish. It is difficult to tell the name of a particular animal to purchase first, but there are a few factors that should be considered before selecting animals for your livestock. You should consider your ability and passion for caring for these animals. If you have plenty of space, you can select more than one animal. At a limited space, laying hens will be a good choice. To get yarn, you can raise fiber animals and sheep. If you are scared of larger animals like sheep, you can select angora rabbits.

An urban homesteader should consult limitations and restrictions by town government before keeping animals in your house. Keep it in mind that livestock requires regular care and you have to feed all animals twice a day. You should have sufficient time and resources to feed them. You have to make a barn, pens, hay bales and clean stalls. It is important to fill water troughs with fresh water and keep your animals clean and vaccinated.

Getting Started with Livestock

If you are planning to raise livestock, there are numerous preparations that should be done in advance:
Design a suitable fence to secure and separate your house from a farm area. You should collect sufficient details about predators in your area to follow safety precautions to keep your animals safe from them.
You should have plenty of water and food for your animals, even in freezing temperatures.

Prepare a place for animals in advance with all facilities. All things in one place will increase your enjoyment to raise livestock.

Purchase Healthy Animals
You should always purchase healthy animals, such as the eyes should be bright and free from discharge. The animal should be able to breathe smoothly without coughing. The body should not be full of round scars and acne. The animal should have a full body and move freely and easily. You can't buy an animal with swollen legs, joints and mucus coming out

of the nose.

Start with a Chicken Farm

At an initial level, you can start with a chicken farm to get eggs and meat. Chickens work hard for the growth of your farm and they will bring tasty meat and eggs. You can start with popular breeds like Plymouth Rocks, Dominique, and Buckeyes. In your poultry, duck, geese, and turkeys will be a great addition. Ducks can not only give you meat and eggs, but you can raise them to eat unwanted bugs. Geese offer eggs, meat, and feathers. You can keep them on pasture and trim back weeds to protect your farm from predators. Turkey may revive your memory of thanksgiving, but it will be a good addition to your farm. Moreover, you can select sheep and goats. These are intelligent and naughty ruminants to live well with hens. You can make a separate pen for your hens.

Protect Livestock and Poultry from Predators

Your livestock and pets are completely your responsibility; therefore, you should protect them to make predators think that eating them will be harder for them. You can buy a dog like Maremma sheepdog, Akbash, Pyrenees, Komondor, Polish Tatra Sheepdog, Kangal, etc. One of these dogs can protect your livestock from predators like wolves, predator dogs, coyotes, and foxes. It will be good to use physical barriers and protect your animals from predators. You can use light or music in the night to keep predators away from your livestock. It is important to collect information about predators in your area and then deploy right methods to keep them away from your livestock.

Chapter 5: Efficient Space

Making use of whatever space you have may seem like a daunting task. However, there are some really unusual and super cool tricks out there, no matter if you have 5 or 50 square feet with which to work. I will cover the three main types of homesteading so you can grasp the big picture. With each one, it requires a change in mindset, especially if you are a true city slicker. Your old routines will become a thing of the past, especially if you sleep, wake up, go to work, come home, eat, watch TV, go to bed, and repeat. Being a homesteader requires a little bit of ingenuity and work, but the benefits you reap will be completely worth it.

Apartment living can offer a simplicity that takes away the responsibilities of maintaining a yard, and worrying about home repairs. However, you may have to rely on the laundromat for cleaning clothes, and the ease of grabbing take-out food makes it hard to always eat healthy. Becoming a homesteader can not only be a great hobby, but help change your life for the better.

Some easy steps to get you started are listed below, and I will go into greater depth later in the book:

☐ Make use of your windowsills and create gardens! You can plant spices and small quantities of vegetables.

☐ If you have a balcony, create a wilderness of edibles! Container gardens are just as effective in growing vegetables as any other system. There is nothing nicer than seeing a balcony loaded with beautiful plants.

☐ Make your own cleaning supplies. The chemicals used in most in cleaning products can be harmful to the environment and your family. By making your own, you save money and keep a healthier household.

☐ Give up the clothes dryer. String a clothesline outside or if that isn't possible, have a drying rack in your apartment for your clothes. It will save money and energy.

☐ Learn food preservation. All those goodies you grew on your balcony can last you through a winter by learning how to preserve them naturally.

All of these steps can be implemented in your apartment, urban or suburban home. Additionally, there are even more homesteading tips can be used in an urban home, with even a small yard.

In an urban homestead, you have an opportunity to utilize the small space efficiently to create a source of all natural food for your family. Depending on the size of your space, here are some ideas you can implement with even the smallest yard:

☐ Vertical gardening is a huge space saver. You may have seen hanging tomato plants, but pretty much anything that is a vine plant can be grown in a vertical garden. Some examples are peas, beans, cucumbers, even melons!

☐ Beekeeping is a new trend for urban homesteaders because it doesn't require a lot of space to care for the bees and harvest that delicious raw honey.

- Create a homesteader kitchen! Learning how to make your own bread, cheese and other common products you normally purchase at the market will save you money and be very satisfying.
- Compost! This is a key to all natural and chemical free fertilizer. Not only does making your own compost pile save you money, help grow gorgeous vegetables, but it also cuts down on waste at the landfill. Use eggshells, coffee grinds, paper, leaves, grass cuttings and scraps from the table to create your very own compost.

The urban homestead options are a bit broader than the apartment choices, as there is a little more space. However, if you live in a suburban setting, on even just a quarter acre lot, there is so much more you can do!

- Have an egg source – more cities and towns are allowing backyard chickens. They are natural pesticides (they eat ALL the bugs!) and their waste is awesome fertilizer. Check your local town/city codes for guidelines and permits for backyard chickens.

☐ A BIG garden! I am a fan of square foot gardens as they are easy to build and maintain. In Square Foot Gardening by Balal Naeem, there are many tips on it as well as how to build your own 4'x4' box. The great thing about this is you can have as many as you want, depending on space and what other options you want for your homestead.

☐ Goats aren't just for funny YouTube videos... They provide milk and you can make goat cheese (Mmmm!) Of course, goat meat is popular in the Caribbean, another option for your family too.

☐ Rabbits multiply like crazy. I think we have all heard the expression regarding rabbit's reproduction skills... Anyhow, they are a great source of meat for your family. They are easy to breed, and they also require a fraction of the space that a cow or pig would require.

☐ Create a root cellar. This is much easier than it sounds as you do not need a large space, just dig a hole. If you plan to grow potatoes, squash, onions, carrots, or parsnips, this will help keep them for the winter.

As you can see, there is a plethora of ways to create your own homestead, regardless of size of your space. In the following chapters, I will discuss in depth some of these options available to you.

Chapter 6: Poultry And Livestock

Many a times when you buy frozen chicken the piece would be old or spoilt. Inedible you've to throw it. Same goes for other meats also; whereas if you grow your own chicken you can enjoy fresh poultry. Your Homestead can be a haven for chicken, goats, rabbits, cows and other livestock that can help you to eat fresh meat; not to forget the eggs. Having a pen and a cow shed is really a boon for the homestead. Though the cost has to be taken into consideration the returns you get on your investment is well worth a try. It is only initially that you need to buy the chicks, hen and cows. After that they'll multiply and yield for you. Rabbits multiply in numbers and very soon you'll find hundreds of them hopping around your yard. Cows and goats also multiply though not as fast as rabbits or chickens.

Cow's milk

Cow is a God send animal that is of optimum use to us. You can get milk out of cows and that milk can be churned into butter and yoghurt. The flesh of cow is consumed as meat and tastes good. Also cow dung is used as manure/ fertilizer to the soil. It contains antioxidants and is healthy for the soil. You can sell excess milk and cow dung. So a cow is a source of income for you.

Nature is so amazing that there is a use of each and every living being. This is known as the life cycle. For example – chicks eat grains and small worms and parasites that are in your farm. The chaff after removing the grains can be fed to cows as fodder. In case you've a beer factory or sugar mill near your homestead get the molasses from them to feed your cows. They'll yield better quality milk.

Sheep's wool

Goat's milk is also used for drinking and goat meat can fetch you good money. Rearing goats and sheep can also help you to get wool out of sheep. Once winter is over you can shave off the wool from the sheep and set them free for spring. Where as you can treat the wool and make it useful to knit sweaters and winter dresses. The sheep's coat is known as fleece and it is sheered from live sheep. The fleece is washed and dried and then bundled. The entangled pieces are removed carefully and they're categorized to spin as soft or irregular yarn. The wool is dyed in different colors during the manufacturing process.

Poultry

Organic chicken cost a lot more than the normal ones. Yet it is important to eat organic chicken than the poisonous ones that can cause epidemic like Swine flu. Pigs can also be reared in your homestead so that you can eat organic Pork, bacon and gammon and not worry about epidemics. A couple of years ago Swine flu spread like wild fire causing thousands of deaths in the east. It is better to raise your own livestock and be free from sickness.

Organic chicken are tastier and contain less fat. Since they're fresh and from your farm you needn't worry about their quality. The chicken you get in the market is injected with antibiotics and toxic hormones. This is not good for consumption. Grow your own meat and chicks and enjoy organic eggs, chicken, pigs and other livestock.

Sell your excess produce

Organic poultry and other produce will fetch you more money than the usual ones. You can team up with a vendor who will buy regularly from you. This will ensure that you'll have steady income from your poultry and livestock.

Chapter 7: Preserving Your Harvest

Most homesteaders grow more than they need so they can store it for later use, not just because preserved food can last you until the next growing season, but also because it is so darn delicious.

There are many different preservation and processing techniques you can tap into. This chapter covers the most common ones, and they will keep you covered during those not-so-productive, frosty winter days.

Proper Storage

There are fruits and veggies you will want to eat raw and fresh. But you may also decide to can some apples or make an apple jam. For that, proper storage is required. Here is what you need to consider:

Temperature – To prolong the shelf life of your veggies and fruits, they need to be stored in a cool place. That can range between 32 and 60 degrees Fahrenheit. This is crucial, as the right temperature can slow down the multiplying of enzymes, which helps the food decay.

Humidity – The ideal humidity for proper storing is between 60 and 95 percent. That varies for different types of food. For instance, onions don't tolerate humidity over 70 percent, while carrots need it to be between 90 and 95 percent. Ideally, you should have multiple storage places with different humidity levels.

Ventilation – The storage area also needs to have decent ventilation so that warm air doesn't pack inside. Allowing the cool winter air is more than recommended.

If you have a root cellar or even a storm shelter, that will do the trick. Once you make sure that you've got the temperature, humidity, and ventilation covered, make sure to the place is completely enclosed to keep rodents at bay. Your basement is another great solution.

DIY Storage Solution

But what if you have no proper place for storage? Well, you can always create one in your backyard, but it won't be large enough for all of your food. However, you can move closer to off-grid survival with this simple straw-bale trick.

If there is some free space in your yard, you can use it to construct a straw-bale storage box for root veggies such as potatoes, turnips, parsnips, and rutabaga.

Keep in mind that the place should be dry, so don't store in areas where you usually have a lot of snow buildup. Don't place it near your house, either. The straw storage should stay freezing cold on the outside. Here is how to do it:

Place two straw bales next to each other, touching.

Place another two bales parallel to them, about 16 feet away.

Add a straw bale at each end between the bales to enclose the space and make a straw box.

Cover the bottom of the box with a screen so you can protect your food from critters who might dig to get inside.

Add some straw on top of your screen.

Place your roots gently at the bottom. Make sure you don't dump the veggies inside – bumps mean quick spoiling.

Cover the root vegetables with bales of straw, making sure that the box is completely covered.

You now have a breathable, cold storage area.

Fruits and Veggies for Cold Storage

Besides your canned produce (more of that later in this chapter), fruits and veggies can be placed in a cold storage area. If stored properly, they can last you for many months. Here is a guide:

Onions – Most onions will stay fresh for a really long time; however, pick the **good keeper** kind when buying seeds so that they store well. Place the onions in a loose mesh bag. You can even use a pair of stockings – just tie a knot between them. The ideal temperature is
35–45 degrees Fahrenheit.

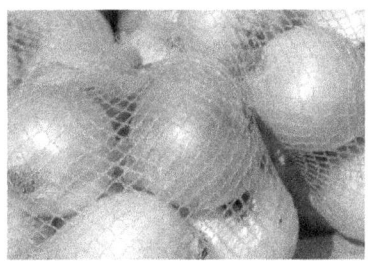

Potatoes – To store potatoes, don't wash them. Inspect well and do not cold store those with bruises. Potatoes keep for a very long time when stored at 32 to 40 degrees, 80–90 percent humidity, and in complete darkness.

Turnips – Don't wash before storing. Trim off the tops and store where the temperature is the lowest. They need about 30–40 degrees Fahrenheit, and high humidity (90–95 percent).

Carrots – For storing, harvest the carrots late in the season and trim off the tops. Store just like turnips.

Beets – Cut off the tops and don't wash the beets. Store just like turnips and carrots – at 32–40 degrees and 90–95 percent humidity.

Tomatoes – You may not have known this, but tomatoes are also perfect for cold storage. The trick here not to store individual fruits, but the entire plant. Also, you don't keep ripe tomatoes – they just have to have a hint of redness. Remove all plants that are still fully green and then pull the entire plant out of the soil. Simply hang it upside down at 55–70 degrees and 60–70 percent humidity. They will ripen over time and you will have fresh tomatoes in a couple of months.

Garlic – Store only when the garlic is completely dry. Tie their tops together in a classic, garlic-style braid. Keep at 30–45 degrees and
60–70 percent humidity.

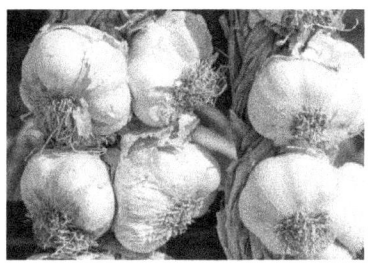

Cabbage – Cabbage stores well, but you need to take a few precautions. First, keep in mind that it is best stored in a slightly damp area – humidity at 80–90 percent and temperature at 32–40 degrees. But cabbage is best stored alone. Why? Because it releases a strong odor that other foods may absorb (think apple with a cabbage flavor). Another thing you need to know is that the longer a cabbage stays in storage, the more intense the flavor when cooked. If you don't like that, you might want to consume it as quickly as you can.

Apples – Apples are perfect for storage as they can easily last you four months, even six. The only thing you need to give them is a temperature of 30–35 degrees and humidity of 80–90 percent.

Pears – Pears are also excellent for storing, but don't pick those that are too ripe and soft as they bruise easily. To keep them healthy, wrap each in a piece of newspaper and store at 30–35 degrees and 80–90 percent humidity.

Freezing

The simplest (and probably the most superior) way of preserving your food is by freezing it. And the best part is that you don't need any special equipment. Chances are you already have what you need around your kitchen.

You can freeze pretty much anything. Some foods may not be so freezer-friendly, but they will still be safe to eat. All you need is to get the temperature right.

It doesn't matter if you have a standalone freezer or a small compartment, the main thing is to freeze at 0 degrees Fahrenheit. Why am I telling you this? Because food that has been frozen at 0 and 10 degrees may look solid; however, there will be a significant difference in the taste. Freeze in rigid containers or Ziplock bags. If using bags, just make sure you press most of the air out.

Vacuum-Sealing

If you have a vacuum-sealing machine, that is the ideal way to prepare your food for the freezer. Thanks to the suction, the air is removed almost completely, which means that the freshness is immediately preserved.

Canning

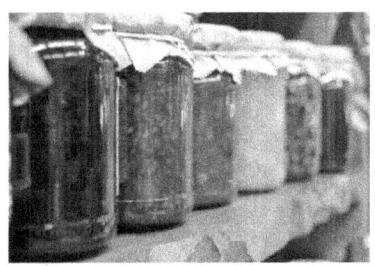

Canning is probably the most popular method of food preservation. Both fruits and veggies can be canned to preserve the flavor and taste. The best thing about canning, though, is that you use the same method for many different things:

Canned pieces of fruits and vegetables
Pickled veggies
Jams and jellies
Fruit preserves
Various condiments like salsa, chutney and relish
There are two methods of canning:
Water-bath canning
Pressure canning

The biggest mistake people make when canning is that they choose a method based on convenience, depending on whether they have a pressure canner at home. But while you can process all foods with each of these methods, some will not be as delicious – or safe to eat. Choosing a canning method depends on the pH level of the food that is being processed:

High-acid foods – most pickled food and fruits, with a pH of 4.6 and lower, should be water-bath canned since this process will destroy the microorganisms that can be harmful.

Low-acid foods – most vegetables with a pH level that is higher than 4.6 should be processed in a pressure canner. This method will destroy even the heat-resistant bacteria found in these foods.

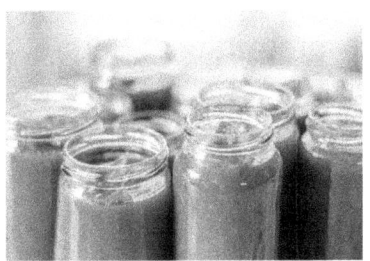

General Safety Tips:
Do not cram the food. Overpacking means that not everything will get processed properly.
Leave enough headspace in the jars – that is the space between the top of the food and the jar's lid. During processing, most foods will expand, so it is essential to give them enough room.
Release the air bubbles. You can do this by stirring the foods within the jar with a nonmetallic spoon or spatula.
Water-Bath Canning
For this method, you need a large canning kettle where you will boil your jars filled

with foods to preserve. Although you can use pretty much any large pot for this method, I advise against it because your jars need to be seated properly for safety and health precautions. Here is how you do it:

Get your equipment ready and clean: jars, lids, screw bands.

Fill the kettle with water, about half to two-thirds up, and start heating until it begins simmering.

Keep everything hot. Place the jars inside the kettle at this point and keep them there for about 10 minutes. Place the lids in another pot filled with hot (not boiling!) water.

Start filling the jar with your prepared food, making sure to leave enough headspace. Also, stir to release air bubbles.

Seal the jars with the lid and add the screw band, making sure it is tightened enough.

Place your jar rack inside the kettle.

Add your filled jars on top, making sure that they are not touching.

Unhook the rack and very carefully lower it to the bottom of the kettle.

Cover the kettle and start timing your processing from the moment the water reaches boiling point. Process for as long as your recipe calls for it.

With a jar lifter, remove your jars from the water. Place on kitchen towels, each jar at about 1–2-inch distance from each other. Let cool completely.

Once they are cool, press the center of the lid to check if you've sealed properly. If the lid doesn't indent, you are good to go.

Remove the screw bands and give your jars a thorough rinse to get rid of any food residue. Pat dry and leave in a cool, dry, and dark place.

Pressure Canning

If you have a pressure canner, then all you need are jars that can be sealed and screw bands. Here is how to do it:

Make sure that everything is clean. Place your jars and lids in a large pot filled with hot water.

Fill about 2 to 3 inches of water in your canner, and preheat it.

Fill your jars, leaving enough headspace.

Release the air bubbles with a spatula that is not metallic.

Seal the jars and tighten with the screw band.

Arrange your jars on the canner's rack carefully, making sure not to touch or tip them. Do not place more jars than your canner's manufacturer recommends.

Close the pressure canner as instructed by the manufacturer.

Once you lock the lid, the pressure canning begins.

Most canners need about 10 minutes for the steam to get released, but follow the instructions in your manual.

Once the processing is done, wait for the pressure to drop to zero, which may take about half an hour. Do not interrupt as this may disrupt the sealing process.

Once your pressure reaches 0, wait for 10 more minutes and then release the pressure, slowly.

Wait 10 more minutes to remove the jars. Place on some kitchen towels, about 1–2 inches from each other.

As previously mentioned, press the center of the lid to check if it is sealed properly. Store in a dark, cool, and dry place.

Important: Do NOT store your jars on top of each other. Stacking applies pressure on the lid that can break the seal.

Drying

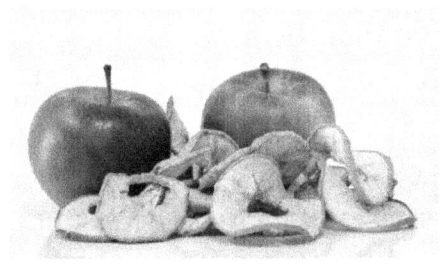

Drying foods, otherwise known as **dehydrating**, is the process of removing moisture from the food to stop bacteria from growing. When drying, the goal is to get rid of about 80–95 percent of the moisture. There are a few factors that can affect your final product:

Heat – The temperature at which you are drying your food is essential – it has to be enough to get rid of the moisture, but not high enough to cook the food. The ideal temperature for drying veggies is 125 degrees Fahrenheit, and for drying fruits 135 degrees Fahrenheit.

Dry Air – You need a dry environment to dry your food. If the humidity is higher, the drying process takes longer.

Circulation of Air – This is also important as the air that circulates absorbs the moisture that the food releases.

The Size of Your Food – For your food to be evenly dried, it has to be uniform in size and thickness.

You can dry your food with a fancy electric dryer (just follow the steps on the manual), in a conventional oven, or by letting it sun-dry.

Oven Drying

Preheat your oven as specified in your recipe.

Arrange the food on your preferred tray.

Place inside and leave the oven door slightly open to let moisture escape.

Dry as stated in the recipe – check for doneness to make sure it is dry.

If you are using trays that have no holes or openings at the bottom, flip the food chunks to make sure they dry evenly.

Sun-Drying

Prepare your food as specified in your recipe.

Place cheesecloth or nylon netting at the bottom of your drying trays.

Arrange the food pieces on the tray.

Cover with another layer of nylon netting or cheesecloth. This prevents insects and dust from getting to your food.

Place the trays in full sunlight.

Check regularly.

Storing Dried Foods

The cooler the air, the longer the shelf life of your dried food. If you store your fruit and veggies at a temperature of 60 degrees (or less), you can expect them to last about a year. If you store them at 80–90 degrees, you will need to consume them within 3 months.

Fermentation

Put simply, fermentation is a process in which microbes such as yeast and bacteria turn the carbohydrates in food into acids or alcohol. If you are making wine or beer, the result will be alcohol. In the case of cabbage, which has acids, you will get **kraut.** It's a nice blend of cooking, science, and magic.

How does it work? Bacteria are introduced to food (like yeast to a dough of bread) and then given the proper conditions to flourish. You can pretty much ferment anything: cabbage, green beans, vinegar, kimchi, salami, yogurt, kefir, and, yes, chocolate.

If you want to dip your toes into fermentation, I suggest you start with making sauerkraut. Sauerkraut is fermented cabbage, and it is made during a process called lacto-fermentation, which is enabled by the beneficial bacteria that are present on the cabbage's surface. All you need is some salt and water. Then you leave the cabbage to ferment in its own brine.

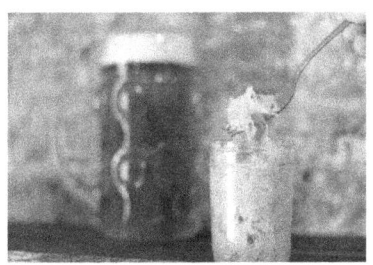

Here's how to make your own sauerkraut:

Cut your cabbage into small chunks and add to a large bucket. Make sure the bucket is not metal as it can react to the bacteria and disrupt fermentation.

Add salt to taste (I use about 1 tablespoon per head, but that's up to you).

Stir well and let the cabbage sit for 5–10 minutes.

Start squeezing with your hands. The squeezing part is what pushes the moisture out of the cabbage. Keep doing this until the cabbage becomes like a wet sponge when squeezed.

The aim is to get the liquid to cover the cabbage completely.

During fermentation, your cabbage will also need to be submerged. You can do this by filling some jars (clean!) with marbles or rocks, and placing them on top of the cabbage.

Cover the bucket with a large towel and tie it off well.

Place the bucket in a cooler place, making sure it is not exposed to a direct light source.

Let it sit for three days and taste. If it is not yet done, return and let it ferment for a few extra days, or until the desired tanginess is achieved. I place it in the fridge at this point.

How long the sauerkraut ferments depends entirely upon your taste. Your kraut is safe to consume at any point.

Making Cheese

If you have a goat, the best way to preserve the milk and stock your fridge with a tasty dairy product is to turn it into cheese. Many newbie homesteaders are intimidated by the cheese-making process. The truth? You cannot really mess it up. And the best part about it? If you get pretty good, making **chevre** can be quite lucrative. If you're not in for the profit, it will cost you nothing but the effort –

which is far less than the price of store-bought goat's cheese.

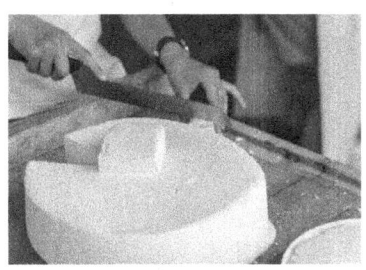

Here is a foolproof way to make it:
You will need:
1 quart goat's milk
2 tbsp white vinegar
⅓ cup lemon juice
½ tsp salt
herbs and spices, to taste
Method:
Grab a colander and place two cheesecloth layers inside.
Heat the milk in a heavy pan until it reaches 180 degrees Fahrenheit. You will need a thermometer for this. Stir occasionally to make sure it is evenly heated.

Remove from heat and stir in the lemon juice immediately.

Add the vinegar, stir to combine, and let the milk sit for about half an hour. Allow to curdle. The curds will not be large, but that's exactly what we are looking for.

Slowly and gently ladle the curdled milk into the cheesecloth.

Add the salt, herbs, and spices. Stir well to combine.

Bring the edges of the cheesecloth together and tie them tightly around the cheese. You can use some kitchen string. I recommend tying it to your faucet.

Let the cheese drip for about one hour.

Untie the cheese, place it on your cutting board, and shape as desired.

Place in the fridge and serve when set. Enjoy!

There are many different ways to preserve the freshness of your food. Try smoking your meat, making juices, vacuum-sealing, and storing in the fridge. Whatever you do, just remember that the fresher your food is when stored, the longer it will last.

Chapter 8: Plan For Making Your Own Backyard Farm

All the things which are made well are all due to the fact that they have been made according to a proper plan. A plan is necessary for constructing and place or thing and similarly constructing your own backyard farm also requires a proper plan which you are required to follow. Do not think that a backyard farm is somehow different from the usual farm as the basic necessities of growing fruits and vegetables seem to be same at every place. Just a proper plan will make your backyard a real success and in making you able to design your own backyard farm where you can grow everything you want without facing any sort of trouble.

One thing which is of worth importance lies in the fact that your plan for making a backyard farm must be well drawn and written so that it can help you out immensely in its designing and construction. Once you make your plan, get stuck to it but do not think that the plan cannot be changed anyways. Once you get a better idea in your mind, you can make amendments in your pre designed plan accordingly

First of all when you plan for constructing a backyard farm in your home, you are required to have a map of your property. If you do not have it already, you can get it from the city planning office which is working near you locally. Once you get the map, make sure that the whole of the topography of your property must be there in your map so that you will better become able to find out what is the path of water which is moving or will move across your land.

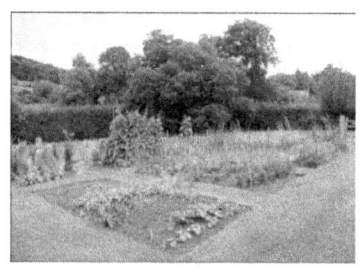

The next step is to look for the placement of different systems which is without any doubt so much critical for the success of each of them. If you are in doubt about the drainage or sewerage system of your house, you are required to hire a professional who will definitely assist you in finding out the solution of your problem. If you haven't done farming before, look out for someone who is expert in urban farming or landscape design so that he may assist you in giving you the right and accurate suggestions according to the availability of place and resources.

You are required to look for the ways by which the better facilitation of appropriate sunlight, water, wind and many other things can be made possible. For this, you are required to completely analyze that how your farm will get the best of sunlight, wind, water, soil and essential nutrients which are required for its proper growth.

In your backyard, you can add different systems like garden, bees, trees of fruits, vegetable plants, chicken and fishes as well. At the first stage of your planning, you are definitely required to work on each system separately and make a flow chart regarding ways of working on all of these systems without facing any sort of problem.

While designing your backyard farm, keep the requirements, curb appeal and privacy in your mind and design the farm accordingly as all of these things will play a significant role in making a perfect design of your farm.

Definitely, you will not want to have an overwhelming work waiting for you at the backyard farm in your home. Instead, you will definitely desire of having your farm to be beautiful and productive. So, in order to make your farm so, you should look for all the possible ways by which the farm can be more and more productive by putting least amount of effort.

Planning a perfect landscape design for your farm is critical so, you should put some extra effort while making a plan for landscaping. Set all the systems in such a way that they not only remain independent but also become able to settle at the same place without any ambiguity.

Plan in such a way that if you also have chicken in your farm, it should remain at a separate place so that they cannot harm the plants of fruits and vegetables.

The hives of bees should be designed so that no bird can harm them. Also, take appropriate steps in saving your plants from attack of birds and several other harmful insects as well.

Take out some time and make a list of all those plants and herbs which you want to be a part of your farm. If you are going to add some herbs, make a plan that how many times a week you will prune them by removing the dead leaves and flowers. Do not forget to add plants after knowing about their exact life span. Plan for adding basil, dill, oregano, mint, tarragon etc. which are excellent to be added to your farm as herbs.

It is for sure that as the likings and tastes of different families vary a lot, there are endless possibilities of farming ideas with all of the families. It is a fact that backyard farming is usually associated with the plans which are highly specific and innately personal. Each family has different needs and innately personal ideas for setting up a backyard helps in finding the exact way by which a particular family wants to have in their own farm. Without any doubt, reconstructing and deconstructing cannot be afforded by everyone as the basic purpose for building a backyard farm through homesteading is definitely to live a sustainable life by cutting down the extra expenses. So, you have to make a better plan all at once but you can change your plan according to the latest plans as well.

But once a plan gets finalized, stick to it and then construct your farm accordingly so that you may avoid any kind of extra costs which will definitely be not liked and afforded by you at all. The most critical aspect of constructing your own backyard farm is to plan about it. So, you should take some of your time here followed by getting some resources which will help you in making the right type of farm and then you can practically implement your plan without getting overboard.

Chapter 9: Types Of Homestead Gardening

The various types of planting are:
1. Square foot gardening
2. Rooftop gardening
3. Container gardening
4. Vertical Gardening
5. Backyard gardening
6. Raise bed gardening
7. Trellis gardening
8. Companion gardening you may also use a combination of these types of gardening as may be needed, based on the kind of plant you choose to grow and the position of your garden space in consideration of other factors such as sunlight, water and wind. Let us take a closer look on each type of gardening and their unique features:

Rooftop Gardening

Land is getting more difficult to find, particularly for planting purposes. Metropolitan homesteaders are thinking that it's hard to grow a nursery due to the absence of appropriate land for planting purposes. Housetop cultivating is probably the best option for metropolitan planters who need to appreciate the incalculable advantages of a nursery in any event, when there is no adequate land accessible for them. Housetop cultivating is particularly useful in metropolitan conditions and urban areas where ground space for garden is rare.

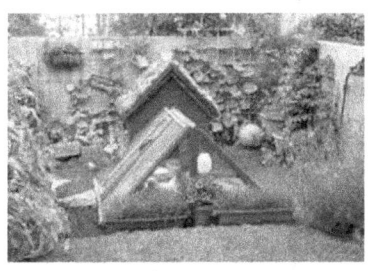

Housetop garden is a man-made nursery space, generally on the top-generally level of a structure picture from Flickr by Jeanne Suliver

This bit of green land can be utilized to deliver products of the soil or just as a play territory — or in any event, for embellishing purposes. Despite the fact that only one out of every odd rooftop top can be changed over into an undeniable nursery, you can utilize the vacant space to grow various foods grown from the ground. You can utilize the whole housetop to make a nursery or plant various natural products, vegetables, spices and blossoms in holders and pots to be set on the rooftops or galleries.

Some housetop gardens don't need inordinate support or upkeep. These housetops function as a straightforward roofing material, and are not proposed for weighty foot falls. Notwithstanding, there are housetop cultivates that need hefty upkeep, finishing, and fortification to withstand the heaviness of the nursery.

Before you begin planting the rooftop, first examine the rooftop and ensure government and natural guidelines permit developing a housetop garden.

See whether the rooftop can withstand the heaviness of the nursery; in the event that it can't, at that point give legitimate fortifications to fortify it.

In the event that you are uncertain of it, counsel a basic architect to get you out.

Pick a plan that contemplates daylight, watering needs, the plants and support.

Recollect you can't develop each plant on your root; so pick the plants astutely after unmistakably understanding its inclination and development capacities.

You can likewise utilize various pots, compartments and grower to assist you with building a decent nursery on the rooftop.

Consider coats to make your nursery less helpless to moving overwhelmed as a result of the breeze.

Likewise consider watering techniques you are going to utilize.

The plants you can develop on your housetop are 'Blue Star' juniper, lavender, daylilies, lady grass, carrots, greens, lemon-pickling cucumbers, shaft beans, lettuce, beats, chives, radishes, and snap peas.

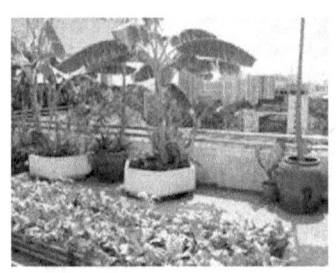

The housetop ought to have the option to withstand the consolidated load of the dirt, the plants, water, and furthermore manage precipitation picture from Flickr by Anne Corbell
Backyard Gardening

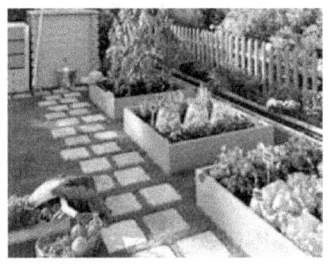

Planting is quick getting one of America's preferred side interests, a period for the entire family to meet up and get grimy! Picture from Flickr by John Cornwell

Everybody longs for a lawn garden — the ideal spot to develop natural products, vegetables, blossoms and so forth! Also, developing your own foods grown from the ground has such an appeal that it is changing over not-the-planting types into — green-thumbs rapidly. There is no age breaking point to take up planting; and you make certain to get enough sun and exercise with cultivating. One of the fundamental strides of lawn cultivating is picking the correct spot to plant your nursery. A portion of the central issues to note while planting your metropolitan homesteading garden are:

Decide the nursery size before choosing what you need to plant. Metropolitan homesteading is tied in with doing you're planting and collecting without anyone else, and naturally. You should ensure that you have the essential devices and time to deal with your nursery. Thus, on the off chance that you are a starter, start little and gradually increment the size of the nursery.

Choose what plants you need to develop contingent upon what you need to devour. Make sure you don't have an excessive number of enormous trees becoming close to your nursery spot, and furthermore imagine future trees

Remember the measure of daylight this spot will get, the breeze and watering needs of the dirt

Plant occasional vegetables and organic products with the goal that you can support the entire year through. Try not to plant a lot of one single plant type; consistently make span plantings of any one vegetable somewhere around at regular intervals or thereabouts. Plants that have short pinnacle periods will in general become quicker, and these can be supplanted right away.

It is likewise acceptable to aggregate plants that have comparable planting conditions and gather dates.

Interplant plants that have a quickly developing time with plants that develop gradually.

Square Foot Gardening

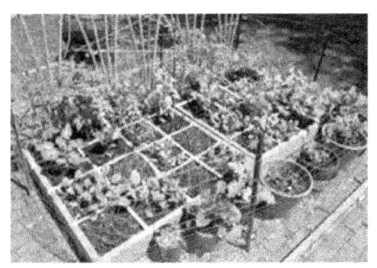

This kind of planting includes the act of masterminding and making pretty much nothing however seriously slept with gardens picture from Flickr by Hans Miller

The training blends ideas from other regular planting procedures remembering a sound concentration for manures, thickly established raised plots and bio-serious concentration to a little, obviously characterized space.

This strategy is especially best for territories with feeble soil, new planters or as procured diversion for individuals with incapacities. It was put on the map by Mel Bartholomew in a 1981 Rodale Press book and succeeding PBS TV programs. You don't generally require a bundle of land to create new veggies.

Offers a simple method to collect a great deal of produce in a little and restricted nursery space. Square foot planting is generally gainful for the individuals who have space limitations and limitations. You will have the option to grow various foods grown from the ground in kept spaces. You can without much of a stretch plant the same number of foods grown from the ground your square foot nursery can hold immediately. To have the option to effectively grow a square foot garden in your home, all you need is barely any feet of land, some great soil blend, seeds and a ton of persistence. Similarly separate the square yard into little pieces in such a way that they can oblige your preferred plants. The accomplishment of square foot cultivating likewise relies upon the daylight, wind, watering, soil blend, composts and the square foot planting boxes utilized.

Before you begin making these crates, you should initially decide the size and area of your nursery. You can buy fabricated boxes however since we are into metropolitan homesteading, constructing square foot cultivating boxes is significant. It is anything but difficult to assemble the crates utilizing fundamental apparatuses. Ensure you assemble an enormous square formed open bottomed box; with segments partitioning the entire box into various littler squares. Presently, fill in this crate with soil blend and begin planting.

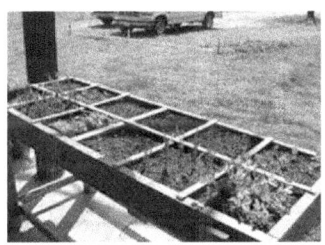

The benefit of square foot cultivating is that you can have a bit of nursery in any event, when you are managing space limitations. You can manufacture a nursery on the housetop or on your front yard picture from Flickr by Vans Devon
Container Gardening

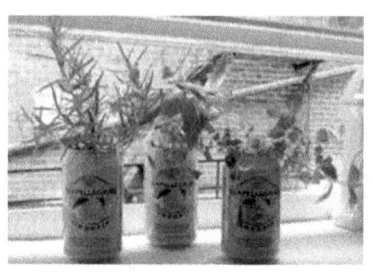

A ton of vegetables develop well even with restricted cultivating space. With a little idea to picking bantam varieties, practically any veggie can be adjusted to thriving in a pot picture from Flickr by Arnstrough

Holder Gardening is another case of good metropolitan estate garden. The very term 'garden' figures out how to summon pictures of lavish green ground garden in the vast majority of us. Be that as it may, for those managing metropolitan space imperatives, having a real estate parcel for cultivating is troublesome. Nonetheless, this ought not put you no longer available for growing a nursery. Compartment cultivating is one of the most effortless and least expensive approaches to have a nursery. You can grow a compartment garden inside, on your housetops, on your entryway patio, on overhangs, windowsills and on your means.

Regardless of whether you incline toward your preferred huge assortment, you may accomplish the equivalent in the event that you furnish it a satisfactorily measured pot with loads of soil and enough water, it will become in any case and prize you with a plentiful reap.

Vegetables that utilization little regions, for example, lettuce, carrots, radishes or plants that produce natural products over an all-inclusive timeframe, for example, peppers and tomatoes are perfect for holder veggie gardens. What you can create in a holder vegetable plot is restricted just by the size of the zone and your creative mind.

Since your veggie plants will make their holders dwelling place, you need to start them off right. Guarantee there is sufficient region for them to form into and pick your dirt and area with care. Here are a few hints for setting up your compartment cultivating for explicit vegetables.

Choosing Containers:

Holders for your veggie nurseries can be:

1.Buckets 2. Bushel containers 3. Window boxes 4. Enormous food jars 5. Nursery pads 6. Old elastic tires cut into equal parts 7.Pails 8. Plastic packs 9. Strawberry pots 10. Washtubs 11. Window grower 12. Wire bins Drainage:

Whatever sort of box you decide for your veggie garden, it ought to have penetrates at the base to permit waste of surplus water.

Color Matters:

Be cautious when taking care of dull colored holders as they will in general assimilate warmth which could harm the foundations of the plants. On the off chance that you utilize dim toned pots, try painting them a lighter shade.

Dimension:

The element of the holder is huge. Bigger veggies like eggplants and tomatoes, requires the utilization of a five gallon holder for each plant. You can build up these plants in two gallon compartments, however you should support the plants widely with more water.

Soil and Fertilizer:

You may utilize top soil in your compartment veggie garden, yet preparing blends would be better. You can pick among vermiculite, peat-based blends or containing peat for your preparing blends. They are moderately sans germ and pH controlled. They likewise grant the plants to get adequate water and air.

Consolidating one segment of fertilizer to two bits of planting blend will upgrade fruitfulness. Applying a total normal compost at preparing will keep your veggies took care of for the entire developing season.

Watering:

Pruned plants consistently need more standard watering when contrasted with that of plants imbedded into the ground. As the season advances and plants create, their underlying foundations will extend and require considerably more water. Insufficient water will make the plants wither. Subsequently, it is ideal to check your pots each day for conceivable requirement for water.

Wind:

The breeze can be an impressive risk for any pruned developed plant and tall veggies, similar to tomatoes, as their top turns out to be hefty when they bear organic products. Attempt to place your compartments in an area where you can deal with the impacts of wind. A breeze will give a decent wind stream and help secure against contagious diseases.

Then again, an amazing breeze can thump down plants and holders. It can similarly tear leaves and make natural products fall. In the event that your nursery is on a rooftop top or raised deck, it is important to manufacture some sort of wind block.

Holder cultivating gives you the opportunity of getting any compartment that you can discover in your lawn and convert it into a plausible and suitable aspect of your compartment garden. Besides, compartment garden gives you the opportunity to move the holders to various areas in your home contingent upon the requirements of the plants. On the off chance that you think your plants will suffocate in the heavy storm, you should simply move that specific compartment inside or to a superior area.

The holder materials you pick will decide plant development, water needs, and daylight. In the event that you are utilizing earthenware or earthen compartments, you need to ensure that you keep the plants soggy as these holder materials will in general assimilate dampness rapidly.

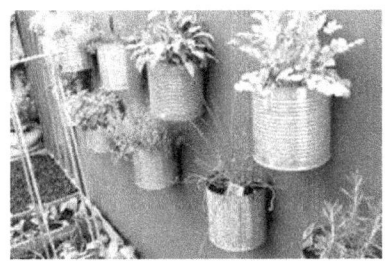

Compartment planting is likewise viable approach to manage awful soil structure, seasons, and weeds picture from Flickr by Marsel Armstrong

Vertical Gardening

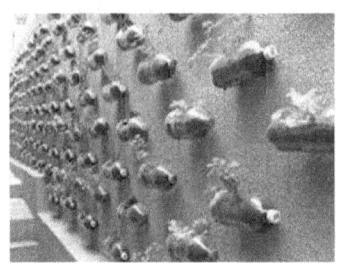

Only one out of every odd one of us has been honored with space to grow a nursery; a few of us need to make with only a divider to call our own. With vertical planting, even a divider is all that anyone could need. Regardless of whether you have a huge divider or only a little pivot to drape a pot on your gallery, you can begin developing upstanding harvests without any problem. With a smidgen of inventiveness and heaps of persistence, you can make an excellent vertical nursery in next to no space picture from Flickr by Reachr

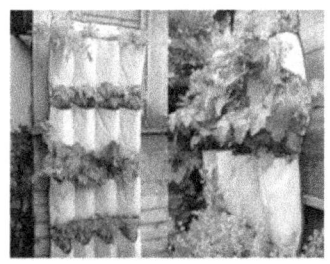

There are different plant assortments, for example, post beans and cucumbers that produce more than twofold their typical yield when you develop them on the privilege measured lattice picture from Flickr by John Mueller

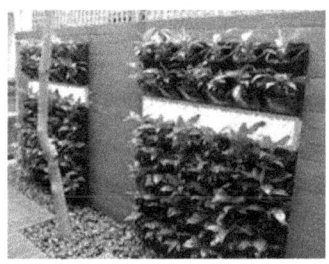

You have crops like tomatoes that develop well and bring a decent yield just when you give them enough help to stand upstanding and off the clammy ground. You should simply give your plants all the

required help, and you can appreciate an awesome nursery picture from Flickr by Sarah Penny

Raised-bed Gardening

Raised bed cultivating is a sort of planting where the earth is framed in 4 foot or 1.2 meters wide beds, which can be of any shape or length. The dirt is raised over the close by soil, inside a scope of six crawls to abdomen high of the rancher, is some of the time encompassed by an edge generally made of concrete squares, wood or rock and might be improved with compost.

The vegetable plants are spread out in mathematical courses of action, much closer together when contrasted with the customary line cultivating. The situating is to such an extent that when the veggies are completely evolved, their leaves just scarcely interact with one another, making a miniature atmosphere in which undesirable plant development is hindered and dampness is protected.

Raised beds produce numerous advantages:

They stretch the planting time frame.

They can diminish weeds whenever orchestrated and planted effectively and decrease the utilization of helpless common soil.

The dirt is free causing the roots to develop effectively as the planter can't stroll on the raised beds.

The close to plant course of action and the utilization of natural manure typically bring about expanded yields in contrast with customary column cultivating and

Abdomen high raised beds causes it workable for the genuinely incapacitated and seniors to develop veggies without the need to twist around to be accountable for them.

Trellis Gardening

Trellising veggies and organic products is a planting strategy that keeps up plants out of the ground, expands creation and usable zone. It likewise ensures your gather, particularly tomatoes, from rotting. There are the same number of trellising decisions as there are sorts to develop.

The mystery is finding or making the most material one for your necessities.

Here are a few yields best for this sort of cultivating style:

Tomatoes

Most tomato varieties profit by a hearty help. Choosing the incredible method to keep up cluttered plants in some type of request is dependent upon the tomato kind and its development plans. Determinate tomatoes are medium-sized plants that create to a lasting full grown measurement and develop all their natural product in a little timeframe.

They are the sort which profits by a little height off the floor zone as enclosures or stakes. Then again, vague sorts keep on thriving constantly, with organic products developing until the plant is harmed by ice or terrible climate. These sorts improve prepared on a lattice framework.

Uncertain tomato assortments frequently develop to gigantic apexes in sweltering climate, subsequently making them very unmanageable. It is just through trellising that the plant specialist can control the branches, empower the daylight to get further into the plant and keep up the organic product uncontaminated.

Trellising likewise permit the plants to be close accordingly coming about to a more powerful utilization of region. Regularly raised tomato assortments include: Big Boy, Brandy-Wine, Early Girl, Honey Grape, Rutgers and Super Sioux.

Pole Beans

Mainstream assortments are Scarlet Runner, Black-Seeded Blue Lake, Kentucky Blue Pole and Kentucky Wonder.

Peas

Sugar Snap and Tall Telephone are the favored assortments on peas.

Melons

Supported assortments incorporate the Blenheim Orange Muskmelon, Delicious 51 Muskmelon, Moon and Stars, and Sugar Baby.

Cucumbers

Armenian and Market-more 76 are the top choices in Cucumber assortments.

Pumpkins and Squash

The exceptionally picked assortments comprise of Jack-Be-Little, Patty Pan and Zucchini Jackpot Hybrid.

The upsides of trellising are not just for tomatoes. Preparing other produce to become upward as opposed to spreading everywhere on over the nursery keeps up the produce off the ground, yet permits you to develop more in a restricted territory. Peas and shaft beans can as a rule reach more than six feet high and are by and large trellised.

Their help can be as plain as a teepee made from willows, a metal control board secured to a metal support posts, or uprights made of wood with chicken link extended in the midst of them. It is ideal to pick a framework reliant on the developing conduct of your supported assortment.

Companion Planting

Companion Planting utilizes zone and draw in accommodating bugs. Numerous additionally concur that particular plant blend have phenomenal and strange forces for supporting each other prosper.

Logical exploration of friend planting has affirmed that some blend have genuine advantages selective to those mixes. Also, viable contribution has shown to a ton of plant specialists how to match off explicit plants for their common worth.

Partner planting works best in:

Assisting each other create as observed by high plants giving shade for sun-delicate littler plants;

Efficiently utilizing garden zone as exemplified by having two plants in a single fix where plant plants spread over the ground while vertical plants develop;

Deterring vermin troubles as common of onions averting a few bugs while some different plants can drive bothers away; and,

Attracting supportive bugs which ordinarily are predators of undesirable creepy crawlies. Valued plant mixes include:

Roses and Garlic

Plant specialists have been developing chives with roses for ages, fundamentally in light of the fact that garlic repulses rose bugs. Garlic chives act simply as anti-agents, yet their little white or purple blossoms toward the finish of spring shows up exquisite with blossoms and foliage of roses.

Cabbage and Tomatoes

Tomatoes are appalling to diamondback moth hatchlings, caterpillars that eat through large gaps in the leaves of the cabbage.

Nasturtiums and Cucumbers

The plant stems of the nasturtiums make it an incredible pal to the meandering aimlessly cucumbers and squash plants. Nasturtiums are known to forestall cucumber creepy crawlies but at the same time are a territory for insatiable bugs like ground bugs and bugs.

Peppers and Pig-weed or Rag-weed

Leaf-excavators favored the undesirable plants to splash plants in an investigation directed at the Coastal Plains Experiment Station in Tifton, Georgia. Simply try to eliminate the blossoms of the weeds before they place seed or you will experience difficulty dealing with the weeds.

Natural ranchers realize that a fluctuated blend of plants results to a sound and stunning nursery picture from Flickr by John Streat

Chapter 10: Gardening Tips And Strategy To Maximize Your Homestead Harvest

The best way to keep high-grade, organically full-grown produce on your table year-around is to grow the maximum amount you can eat, and preserve when your garden isn't producing again. This is often a worthy goal, as home-grown produce, is often more nutritious and delicious than the everyday factory-made fare. In order to make your garden reach its maximum potential, you can implement several growing and conserving methods. As you attempt to produce more organic food, be realistic regarding the time you have got to take care of your garden and manage its harvest, and also ensure you do not more than yourself.

Plan Good Garden Production

Whether you draw your garden plans with paper and pencil or use great vegetable garden Planner, you might still have to think ahead to include these yield-maximizing methods.

1. Start Early, End Late. Use tunnels, cold frames, cloches and different season-stretching devices to maneuver your spring dish season up by a month or more. In fall, utilize row covers to shield fall crops from deer and frost but postponing the harvest period for a large variety of cold-tolerant root as well as greens crops.

2. Emphasize What Grows Well for You: Crops that are not difficult to grow in one climate or soil sort could be large challenges in others, therefore aim to repeat your successes. For example, my carrots are rarely spectacular however my beets are strong, therefore I keep carrot plantings minimised and grow several beets my sufficient for my family. After you realize vegetables that stand out in your garden, growing more than enough your family is a huge step closer to food self-sufficiency. You should not overlook the knowledge of your fellow homesteaders.

3. Grow High-Value Crops: "Value" is subjective, although growing things that will be expensive at shops is quite sensible, provided the crops suit your climate. Hhowever, value could also be about flavor, which could mean earmarking area for your favorite tomato varieties and herbs first, and then considering the amount of cash you could save by growing other crops.

4. Grow the "Shoulder Season" Fruits: You could always choose and stash early raspberries and June bearing strawberriess in the freezer before your garden's vegetables take over your kitchen. Raspberries that bear within the fall and late-ripening apples are less likely to contend with summer-ripening vegetables for your food preservation time.

5. Grow Good things to Drink: Asides, growing what you eat, also grow tasty beverages. I permit rampant apple mint to cover a hillside as a result of it being a good tea plant, and rhubarb stalk tea makes a tart substitute for lemonade. Can or freeze tree fruits and juices of berries,

or create them into soda, alcohol or wine. Recently, well produced blueberry, strawberry, including apple wines start at $12 a bottle, therefore knowing how to make yours, can yield more income.

6. Plant Perennials. Edible plants that come back yearly save planting time, and maintenance is restricted to annual fertilising, weeding and mulching. Rhubarb and Asparagus tthrive wherever winters are cold, sorrel is a terrific perennial green, horseradish and grow almost everywhere and gardeners in climates with mild winters grow bunching onions or perhaps bamboo shoots as perennial garden crops.

7. Opt for High-Yielding Crops and Varieties: Few things are more heartbreaking than nurturing a tomato plant for 3 months only to reap 3 fruits from it. Don't let this happen to you! Network with local gardeners in search of varieties well-known to grow well in your area, or see our list of the most effective regional varieties, and try them. Keep your mind open to historically bred hybrids, classic as well as superior open-pollinated

varieties. With sweet peppers, as an example, several gardeners want the quick maturation of hybrid varieties and their disease resistant to make a good crop. The opposite is true with vegetables such as, peas, lettuce, beans, winter squash and others that do not need hybridization to make them more productive.

8. Include Essential kitchen Herbs: After we conducting our online mega-survey of the most effective garden crops, several gardeners told us about the rewards of growing culinary herbs like dill, mint, basils and parsley, that are not difficult to grow yet expensive at shops.

9. Don't grow too much of the same thing: Last year, some friends who had not gardened in a while told me they had spent the weekend planting fifty tomatoes and pepper plants. Wow! At my house, fourteen tomato plants as well as ten peppers offer the 2 of us one year's source of driedd, canned and frozen treatt — including extras to give away. Growing more would be a waste of your space, time and precious soil resources. Unless

you sell at a farmer's market stand, aim to grow solely as much as you can use.

10. Try something new annually: A fun part of gardening is discovering new things, and only a few have ever grown several edible crops worth trialing in gardens. Keep in might that you will need to try cool-season crops in both fall and spring before deciding whether or not they are garden-worthy. Some crops (or even varieties) that are dud if cultivated in spring could amaze you with their exuberance if grown in fall.

Use space with efficiency

It is a rare gardener who has enough fertile growing area as he or she would love, and most gardeners work limited-space gardens as intensively as we can. (Read tips on how to "Make the most of small or Shady Gardens.") In gardens of any size, attempt these tips to make prime use of every bed and row.

11. Plant in Blocks: According Colorado State extension service analysis, you can quadruple per-square-foot production of small kitchen vegetables like carrots,

lettuce and beets by planting them in blocks within wide beds instead of in rows. Block planting makes economical use of space by eliminating unnecessary pathways and keeping the spacing between plants tight.

12. Try vertical Gardening: After moving from suburban Baltimoreto a ground-floor condo in Albuquerque, N.M.Ary Bruno a lifelong organic gardener went vertical to make maximum use of his space. By adding three to four inches of compost to his compact beds every spring, Bruno can grow pole beans, trellised tomatoes and cucumbers in his patio garden in summer, followed by greens in fall. Vertical growing will greatly increase your garden returns.

13. Interplant Friendly Crops: "I plant lettuce plus spinach when planting a seasonal crop such as tomatoes, to grow inside the shade of the higher plants," says a renowned farmer

14. Succession Sow for Steady Harvests: With snap peas, sweet corn, lettuce and other vegetables that mature like clockwork, build 2 sowings 3 weeks apart

to lengthen your harvest season. Or, plant 2 varieties with totally different maturation times on the same day.

15. Use Seedlings to Run Tight Successions: Let's say it is June, and you would like to replace bolting lettuce with summer squash. If you had thought ahead and commenced squash seeds in containers, you could pull out the lettuce, plug in squash and add some compost, all in the same afternoon. Seedlings usage tightens up the timing of succession planting (sometimes known as "relay planting"), whether or not you replace spring spinach with fall broccoli or following cucumbers with fall snow peas sprouting indoors.

16. Plant One New Edible weekly: Feeding squash daily can get old, but, you wouldn't have that contains if your garden offers small bites of unusual veggies, like bulb fennel, bok choy, escaroles, celeriac, radicchio and white beets. I like to devote 1 wide row to "this-and-that" crops that I sow small pinches. Organizing the garden using the method, gives me a place to try

unfamiliar veggies and keeps these crops from getting lost.

Smarter Garden harvest home

Growing a great crop is just half of the story. As every crop comes in, you will need to pick, cook or store your fresh vegetables with a constant eye towards flour preservation, good eating qualities and nutrition.

17. Pick Things at Their Peak: Look forward to harvesting in the morning, which is when plants are plumped up with moisture and nutrients. Preserve the nutrition and flavour of leafy greens, root crops and lots of different vegetables by refrigerating them, however don't chill storage onions, sweet potatoes, tomatoes or shallots.

18. Grow Cut-and-Come-Again Crops: Chard is that the best example of a vegetable that bounces back on every occasion you harvest a few leaves and stalk, and lots of different vegetables will make a second or third comeback if given an opportunity. If cut high, broccoli, cabbage and even bulb fennel can grow

little secondary heads, and bush beans that you just keep picked (harvesting gently, using 2 hands) often produces 3 flushes of pods and blossoms. Look for cut-and-come-again lettuce varieties, also.

19. Pick early and often. Several garden vegetables get harvested when they are technically immature— budding heads of broccoli flowers, barely plump snap peas or tender very little summer squash. At times, quick harvesting assist the vegetable plants in reproduction stage stays stretched, and in turn increases harvest. In a study from the University of American state Extension comparison summer squash which is harvested daily as baby squash with some other varieties picked every 2 to 3 days, researchers gathered more twice as many baby squash from the plants which were more intensively harvested.

Limit Inputs of time and money

What's keeping you from growing a much bigger garden? For several individuals answer is, a bigger garden would take more energy, money andtime. Do not let such hindrances stand in your way! You can make your garden less hungry for time and supplies in eight ways.

20. Use Free Fertilizers: make use free, nitrogen-rich fertilizers such as, human urine and grass clippings. You can mulch crops with chemical-free grass clippings, or create a chemical tea by steeping clippings in water. Dilute one-parturine with twenty parts of water, and use the tea produced within the garden and to feed seedlings. For more info and liquid fertiliser recipes, you could check out Free, home-made Liquid Fertilizers.

22. Save Seeds: Saving little quantity of your own seeds will certainly mean less expenses on your garden every year, and you will enjoy the convenience of continually having a ready supply of plant seeds on hand. Begin with superior open-pollinated varieties, and work with vegetables that are usually harvested when dead-ripe, such as melons, tomatoes, dry beans and winter squash.

23. Weed Early and often: Most garden crops need weeding a minimum of 3

times: plan to weed 5 to 7 days when transplanting or sowing, once more 7 to 10 days later, and a third time 3 to 4 weeks after the crop has been planted. By then, the plants ought to be sufficiently big to mulch and should have lots of leaves to shade the soil's surface.

24. Make and Use Your Own Compost: Youu will still be compelled to get high-quality organic compost, however, create a habit of piling together tattered mulches, leaves, pulled plants and different organic materials to form a rich compost at no cost. Additionally, use a worm compost bin or an enclosed composter to capture your kitchen garbage.

25. Grow Your Own Mulch: If you run out of leaves and grass clippings before your garden has been adequately mulched, think about adding sorghum, an annual summer grain, or you could introduce a sorghum-sudan grass hybrid (also known as "sudex") to your mid summer planting plans. These crops will grow to six feet high or more in sixty-five days, and the

huge plants create huge mulch if pulled or cut down just before they set seed.

26. Naturalize with helpful Plants: Last year, after running a story on self-seeding crops, several readers wrote to inform me concerning their perpetual planting of winter squash and pumpkins. If allowed to grow in compost piles along the fence, butternuts and different winter squash varieties makes themselves so at home thereby, becoming a permanent garden feature with work from the gardener. Of the thirty-foureasy, self-seeding crops we named; cilantro, calendula, winter squash and pumpkins received the most fan mail.

27. Use the proper Tools: you can create garden with just a shovel; however, the work would be far more economical and enjoyable if you utilize tools that suit you and your garden. Hoes and long-handled spades that you can use while standing is best a large garden. However, small tools should be considered if you work in small raised beds. Whichever style you use keeping a sharp edge on all your hoes and spade would always make them work

better. If you are a female gardener and notice that the grip, size and style of garden tools you have tried within the past do not suit you well, Green Heron Tools sells cool gardening tools designed mainly for women.

28. Water as efficiently as you can: Water, being a precious resource everywhere, no gardener can afford to waste it. For watering summer crops like peppers, okra, sweet corn and tomatoes, mulches and soaker hoses are very helpful. Water can also be captured in rain barrels and route to garden beds making use of perforated soaker hoses. Learn more concerning wise watering.

Plan to stock up

Part of maximizing garden returns is being diligent about usage of everything you grow, and since several crops ripen in large flushes, home food preservation is that the best way to control food waste. Like growing a garden, food preservation is a talent best learned over many seasons as you attempt completely different methods and recipes. Although you buy seasonal products from local organic farmers instead of planting them yourself, you could still be in control of your food supply by preserving.

29. Grow Crops That Store Themselves: As long as they are handled gently and given time to cure, garlic, dry beans, onions, winter squash and sweet potatoes can be kept for months in a cool, dry place — no processing needed. Growing types that store for a long time, like shallots and butternut squash, would enable you to eat fresh food from your garden all winter.

30. Build a Root Cellar: Crops storage in a passively cooled basement Root cellar is undoubtedly one of the best ways to preserve food. you can make one yourself by following these plans for a DIY root cellar.

31. Freeze in small Batches: Some garden produce would go to waste if you freeze extras in small batches every few days. For instance, add green beans, cubed summer squash, chopped peppers, sweet corn or pesto containers or small scalable bags and toss them in the freezer. You could

also try mix-and-match bags of similar vegetables, like chopped kale with chard. Freezing is less technical than canning, with fewer limitations on how veggies can be combined. Add packets of veggies to pastas, soups or other dishes.

32. Learn how to can: one of the easiest and most popular method to put by food is water bath canning, this involves submersing jars stuffed with home grown goodies — like tomatoes sauce, pickles, tomatoess, relishes, jellies and jams— in mere boiling water. This method has a delightful finality to it, as several properly canned foods last for over a year. In my experience canned pickles are best consumed within a year, however, cannedpears and tomatoes sauce are as good after 2 years as they are after one. This implies if I finish the winter, with an excess of, say, tomato sauce, I cut back a tomato plant or 2 in the coming year's growing plan. Although you don't grow your own produce in your garden, canning may be a helpful talent to find out, enabling you to use sseasonal fruits and

vegetables once they are abundant at local farmers markets.

33. Network without charge Pickings: Go browsing to find organic gardeners and farmers with excess turn out on their hands. Native Freecycle teams will assist you notice individuals with unpicked apples or blemished pears, otherwise you will use native e-bulletin boards to arouse what you would like. If you've got friends or relatives United Nations agency grow massive gardens or have mature fruit trees, raise them to decision you once they have an excessive amount of one thing.

34. Trade for What You Don't Have: If you've got associate degree abundance of one thing extraordinary, trade with somebody United Nations agency has one thing else. In Louisa County, Va., Glenda Maphis used this strategy to assist her family garden feed 5 kids. "Here and there we'd would like one thing that we have a tendency to couldn't grow, like corn," Maphis says. "We'd trade a bushel of inexperienced beans for corn from our

dairy-farming friends, and are available home with milk from their vat, too. Jelly became a true item for U.S. to trade. We'd typically trade the jelly for cherries, conserve, inexperienced apples for pies, chicken feed, fodder and smoke-dried meats."

35. Try Drying: Among self-sustaining gardeners, there is a trend toward drying as a food preservation methodology. Once you dry fruits and vegetables in an exceedingly an electrical dehydrator or star dehydrator (or in the sun with arid climates), they take up a lot of less area and keeping their shelf quality for several months under great conditions. You need not worry regarding losing your food as a result of broken freezer or a blackout, and cooking with dried mushrooms, celery, peppers and tomatoes is oh-so-simple. To confirm you do not lose dried product to bug invaders or an excessive moist, properly store them in airtight containers.

36. Take Stock in Late Winter: Before you planting spring garden, take adequate stock of what you have got left in the deep

freezer, root cellar and in dried batches. Did you run out of a particular stock in December that you were yearning for in January and February? Do you have items left, and are not certain whether or not you will be ready to use them up? Take notes of what you want more, and what you do not really need in the forthcoming year, and adjust your garden plans accordingly.

Chapter 11: 10 Easy Ways To Grow Plants For The Beginning Edible Landscape Gardener

If you're thinking of or planning to start a garden or consolidating delicious plants into your landscape, start with some effortless, easy-to-grow, tried, and true fruits and vegetables to help secure a successful harvest. Here's a list of ten fruits and vegetables that are not only fairly effortless and easy to grow, but they are also well-appreciated by a lot of people and have lots of culinary uses.

1. Carrots - Make a very impressive addition to landscape beds with their vibrant, fern-like foliage. Carrots are root crops and are regarded as cool-weather vegetables. They will withstand light frosts, making them pleasant for late fall and early spring. Beyond the orange carrots, we usually see in the market; you can also grow white carrots, yellow carrots, and purple carrots. Seed records offer various sizes, shapes, and colors, including purple, white, red, and yellow.

2. Lettuce - Like the carrot, lettuce is also a cool-weather vegetable, although new, more heat-tolerant classes are being developed all the time. I've found leaf lettuces to be the most straightforward to start within the garden or backyard. And the many colors, leaf shapes, and forms make leaf lettuce a great boundary addition to the edible landscape. What I like best about leaf lettuce is the cut, come back, cut, and come again characteristic. As you cut the leaves you need, more will grow until it gets too warm and the plant fades (flowers and goes to seed).

3. Peas - Peas are a garden snack meal in my family. My children love it. Very few really make it into the home and to the table. Like pole beans grown on poles, they need a frame or something to climb, but they are a bit smaller and don't look to require the same sturdiness that the bean plants do. I've very favorably used chicken wire or tomato cages or a bit of for the plants to climb. When set against a fence, these make very attractive additions to the landscape with their fine flowers and pretty leaf and plant edifice. You can get started with peas by immersing them in water for a couple of days before planting to soften the seed's outer layer. Peas are a more chilling weather vegetable, but you can prolong their growing period by starting in part shade (free from much sun) where the sun won't beat down on the plants for lengthened periods.

4. Radishes - Radishes are often prescribed as a vegetable to start with for children's gardens because they are such a quick, easy-growing root plant. Just follow the directions on the seed packet, and you'll have radishes for your salad in less than four weeks! For the best taste, grow these in colder weather (40-70 degrees is perfect).

5. Cucumber - A not-too-cold-weather, full-sun vining plant, cucumbers are easy to start from seed—plant on slopes in full sun. The heirloom, lemon cucumber, is as straightforward to grow as the more traditional cucumbers you see in grocery stores. If you have confined space, make sure you have a frame that the vine can climb. Or, try one of the small varieties and grow in a vessel.

6. Basil - A great plant to grow and experiment within the kitchen. This herb is available in various varieties with diverse colors, textures, and tastes, including cinnamon basil, lemon basil, sweet basil, purple ruffles basil, and many, many more. The sweet-smelling leaves are used in salads and can also be used fresh or dried to add flavor in stews, poultry, meat, vegetables, vinegar, pesto, and pasta dishes.

Basil is a yearly plant that can be planted in a variety of garden settings. Grow them in the nursery(garden) or, if you don't have a lot of space, they make exceptional potted plants placed on kitchen windowsills for easy gathering when cooking.

7. Beans - Like basil, there are many beans to choose from to grow in the home garden. However, I suggest a bush bean for beginners because pole beans grow on a vine and require a trellis or something they can climb. This may not be something you're willing to invest time or money into it if you're commencing. Beans are simple, effortless, and easy to start from seed, and if you want to jump-start them, immerse them in some water for a couple of days before planting them in the garden. This will weaken the outer shell of the bean, which speeds germination. Kentucky Blue is a great pole bean while Blue Lake is a common bush-type green bean. Both are delightfully plucked right from the garden.

8. Sunflowers - Do you know you can grow sunflowers for the seeds to roast for snacks or serve to the birds throughout winter? This plant is incorporated in this list because their sunny faces make a pleasant addition to the garden landscape and because they are easy to grow and give a tasty seed. Additionally, sunflowers attract bees, which are a necessary part of a healthy garden. Begin sunflowers from seed in full sun, water always, and appreciate the view.

9. Tomatoes - Do you know while tomatoes have prominence for being a bit more challenging to grow, if you retain a few things in mind, you'll find that they're a very pleasant plant that is effortless to grow and doesn't take all that much extra effort? Tomatoes like it not-too-cold (warm), so be sure to pause until after the last cold in your area to set them out quickly and plant them in a bright and sunny area that is also warm. Try them facing the house where the heat circulates the plant. Improve the soil you plant tomatoes in with compost to ensure the plant gets the nutrients it needs from the soil. Lastly, water regularly and intensely. If you see any indications of disease you don't appreciate, take immediate action quickly. Your best bet is to contact your local extension or renowned nursery for advice. Take photos and samples of the diseased part of the plant so the local experts can present the best advice possible.

10. **Strawberries** - This sustained fruit is a dreadful addition to a delicious landscape.

They make great decoration plants or ground cover with striking foliage, attractive white flowers, which are followed by sweet and delicious red fruit that is perfect for the taste bud. Plant one type or all three (I will mention) of the following types to maximize the growing season. Day-neutral strawberries produce berries during the growing season; Ever-bearing berries which produce two-three crops intermittently during spring, Summer and Fall. Finally, June-bearing which produce one crop over two weeks in the spring; however, the day-neutral berries tend to be smaller than June-bearing types. Because Ever-bearing and day-neutral types produce fewer runners than June bearing strawberries, they are excellent for growing in vessels or gardens with restricted space. Strawberries are a full-sun fruit and fancy a sandier soil.

Chapter 12: Raising Chicken

RAISING CHICKEN:
- *Egg and meat productions*
- *Dual purpose breed*
- *Housing your flock*
- *Raising day-old chicks*
- *Bedding area*
- *Temperature requirement*
- *Water requirement*
- *Predator protection feeding*
- *Health concern*
- *Coccidiosis and parasites*
- *Respiratory problems*
- *Bird flu*

RAISING CHICKEN

When properly raising chickens for eggs is handled, it should not be hard at all. Everything you need to do most is to create and operate a proper coop. Your chickens can yield the greatest amount of eggs if they know they live in a safe, secure, and spacious climate.

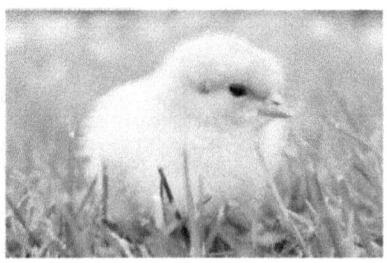

Select a breed that is in line with your purpose

There's numerous dozens as well as dozens of popular chickens breeds, ranging from of the gigantic Jersey Giants to the quail-sized petite bantams. Most are gorgeous, and others are less beautiful but incredibly good at what they're doing (making meat or eggs). So several chickens are extremely good at foraging a massive proportion of their food and thus are colored to prevent predators from capturing it. Others are brightly colored and much more "domestic" disposition.

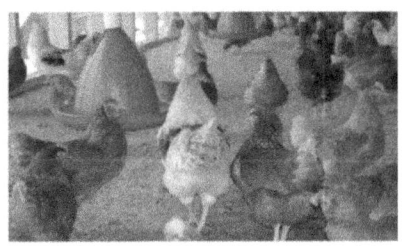

MEAT AND EGG PRODUCTIONs:
Egg production
Unless you don't plan to eat many of your chicks and just want eggs, and lots of

them, realize one of the egg-laying breeds. The most famous of these is the White Leghorn. Leghorn hens are lightweight and healthy and appear to be a little flighty. And they do lay eggs; It isn't unusual to get over 300 eggs a year to a good hen.

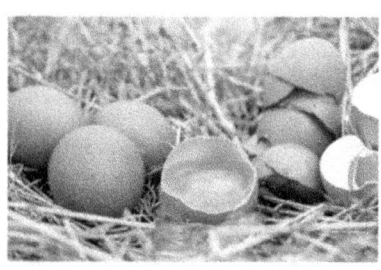

Are you looking for a prettier color than pure old white? Search just in a catalog of poultry to find a better-looking breed that lays a lot of good eggs, though. Many of the top egg-layers in development lay white eggs but are lighter hens.

Meat production

I raised hundreds and tons of chickens, but the white Cornish Rock crosses much outweigh everything else you would purchase for the sheer feed conversion aspect. You could go from tiny chicks to tall, butchering-sized birds in much less than two months. We start raising these, but these birds dress up like youthful turkeys at three months.

Dual Purpose Breeds:

All right, do you want anything from beef to eggs? There are many so-called dual-purpose types. Such fabrics are more substantial than lightweight, and there are also loads of soft brown shells. You won't get the crazy quick turnaround as you do with the Cornish Rock variants with a butchering bird, but instead, you will let the hens hatch their eggs and collect the chicks.

I managed to save some Cornish Rock hens from the breeders, aiming to add a broad scale to my flock. It's not running suitably.

Its legs are its weak spot. They usually experience sore feet or broken muscles sooner or later. And they head down there, and they can't even walk.

There are several various rare and special breeds available, and several of them I have bred. Not only do you get your chicks, but you can market the leftover young birds or breeders at a reasonable price to many other hobbyists. My children always had numerous chickens as 4-H ventures when they grew up. And they'll pick up both these prospective consumers for their purebred chickens through the use of the 4-H A homesteader as well as the county fair.

You could also choose among more substantial "standard" breeds with these "spiffy" breeds, such as the different colors of feather-footed Cochins and also mop-headed Polish to tiny Mille Fleur panties that also fit in your hand. Only take a list of the poultry and check the range. In addition to searching (but also drooling over) poultry catalogs, you can also visit poultry breeders in one area as well as attend poultry swaps as well as fairs to understand about or see various breeds in "person."

How Many Chickens do you need:

We also prefer to overdo when purchasing chicks or chickens. That is not a good idea, particularly for poultry beginners.

With a dozen hens on eggs, a family of five will do very well. When you find you need more eggs for a bit, then you can still add a couple more hens. This leads to fewer accommodations, chores, feed, and space.

Sure, you want to collect some chickens with both eggs and later butcher. Why not continue with 25 chicks, got a bunch of fancy ones to have fun? Those small chicks take little space, feed, or work. Then then, as they hit maximum capacity, they swarm a smaller coop and suck every week a 50-pound bag of grain.

Housing your flock

There's no chance you should hold the chickens.

Luckily, chickens are the most comfortable homegrown livestock to take care of.

How big is the Coop? A dozen hens snugly fit in a coop with 8'x10'. It helps them to roost quarters, sleep and get their food and water while being free to race about and search and scratch as chickens want to do.

Going to raise day-old chicks

You always either go over to the feed store to order or rent, your baby chicks or lease them. But you'll pick them up in the post office when you order them from a catalog. Mail order chicks in brief, sturdy cardboard boxes to holes inside them continue to come up for airflow—sturdy cardboard boxes with holes in them. Food or drink is not required as day-old chicks only survive off the nutrients absorbed from the shell. But as they get home, they feel thirsty as well as hungry.

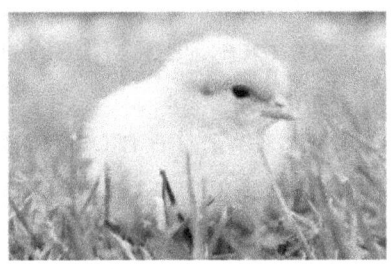

These delicate babies require four things: a safe, dry, draft-free brooding area, warmth from a source of heat so they can stay warm sufficient (hot air temperature isn't enough; they need to have a temperature of 92-95 ° F at first), feed, as well as water.

Bedding area:

At first, Bedding should be a newspaper for fresh chicks. If you render shavings down, they can consume more shavings than feed. I told you at. First, they weren't too intelligent. Consider replacing the newspaper when they have already eaten well with wood shavings and or ground corn cobs. Don't use or they'll eat sawdust. It is very dusty and can cause problems with breathing. With meat breeds, leaving the newspapers down for just one day is a good idea. These chicks are more significant and still have thin bones and muscles. As their feet slip as well as their legs spray onto the slick surface of the papers, they can create leg problems.

So after four weeks, and then when the chicks are feathered out, you will begin shifting them to their young adult house, finalizing with roosts. Roosts should be stepped up for these young birds, so that they should hop up on the bottom echelons, then on to the more robust tiers they prefer. It isn't going to be long until they just float off to the roof. Chickens prefer square material to rounded roosts, but it's simple to create on their feet.

You can buy boxes of metal nests, or end up making your own. I

Had relatively stable luck with a rear, edge, as well as top plywood and 1 "x 12" spacer timber

I like one's boxes, comprehensive as well as high around afoot, and about 18 inches deep. This is big for a little hen, but it's comfortable for a big hen; as such, your boxes will be versatile.

The side of your nesting box tier has to be sharply sloped towards the giving up to stop chickens roosting mostly on nesting boxes. Position a 1-inch pole along the front of the boxes few other inches, and a hen will even fly up, land on it, and choose the bundle she wants. As a result, it results in fewer "arguments" over nests and fewer broken eggs.

Temperature Requirement:

So if you carry your chicks back for the first time, make sure they sustain 92-95 ° F in their brooding area. This is the first week that should be kept up. You should then reduce the temperature by 5 ° per week till you're at 70 ° F, as well as the chicks, are well-feathered.

Using a red heat lamp is better than having a clear one. It will often keep picking up. Calling is if the other bird's peck one or even more chicks. They 're going to begin pulling feathers, but get viciously worse once the poor chick is a horrific mess or either their pen mates hunt and kill him.

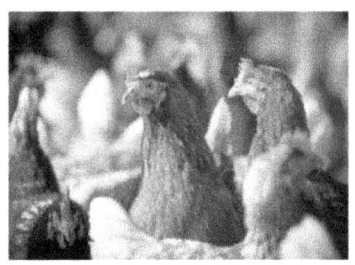

If this begins to happen as well as watching closely, spread the particular grass as well as bits with fruit and in a cage, put some pine tar mostly on a pecked creature, as well as dim the lights. It can also be accomplished often by attempting to hang a sack over one or maybe more windows.

If they keep focusing on the one bird, you're going to have to delete it or destroy it. You can put it back after the feathers regrow, and they'll usually leave it alone.

Picking is indeed a sign with too hot or too cluttered chicks, so avoid such situations. Preventing picking is simpler than curing it! s If you dote your chicks in a small house, near one corner, you can hold a heat lamp first from the ceiling.

Making a cardboard circle a foot tall, and 6 feet in diameter is a good idea. It contains the fresh (not so smart!) Chicks corralled by fire, but safe to run away from it if they so choose a wish, and also near to food and drink.

When you're using some other device instead of a hot lamp but also a field brooder, it's a smart move to have a tiny light at night. The chicks are prevented from throwing themselves into a corner and smothering each other.

I had such problems with our home-built kerosene brooder on our Montana mountainous region homestead because we immediately placed a kerosene lamp onboard often at the edge of both the brooder pen and even stop driving. I used a vacant stock tank as well, and it works pretty well, you should put a heat lamp, leaving the middle with the food and clean water for a more relaxed place.

FEEDING:

The industrial chick-starter is usually the cheapest feed to use.

It is crumbled grain, neither too thin, nor too coarse, supplying vital nutrients to keep them developing quickly.

"But what happened to Grandma? I can assure you Grandma fed her chickens on a combination of good cornmeal, oatmeal, milk, and hard-boiled eggs. She, therefore, messed things up so that it rendered a crumbly dough-like feed as well as feeding them many times a day, leaving in just enough their pan, so they had little left at next feed.

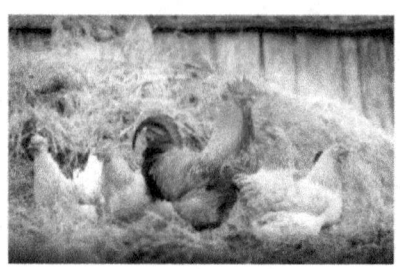

(To keep it from sculpting), but they weren't going to wait too long for the next meal. Also, note Grandma didn't have to train those super-duper Cornish Rock combination chicks either. They are moving so quickly they have unique requirements for feed. Some have no feed remaining 24/7 in front of them; otherwise, they can cause knee issues, as well as being unable to move and suffer.

You can have the stream they will consume in a day for each of these broiler chicks, then have it flow out at night time, as well as fill throughout the feeders again in the morning.

WATER REQUIREMENTS AND PREDATOR PROTECTION:

WATER REQUIREMENT:

You'll need to have a 2-foot long chick feeder as well as a two quarter watering container for every 25 chicks. Chicks are quite susceptible to flooding, so when they're small. When you just position a bowl of water, and you lose a couple of babies in such a brooding field for sure.

Almost as soon because you get your chicks to box in, spend the effort to dip each chick's beak and in water so they'll know how to drink but where the water is. This is also a good reason to place 3 Tbsp in for the first three days.

Stay active. Be active. It makes them off well. New or unique chick vitamin packages, minerals, as well as electrolytes are available to assist get the babies going. Typically, we have this, too. Hold sure feeders complete (excluding the broiler chicks at night).

It's amazing how fast baby chicks could even dehydrate to death and can hunger. Chicks require grit to digest their meal, in addition to feed and water. Sprinkle that little grit regular on the meal. Do not use a ton, or they are going to consume the food, not the meal.

PREDATOR PROTECTION

All have a story about a "fox who got my chickens." And that we have only lost one designed to set hen to a predator in all of the years we've lived throughout wild and isolated land. So this is not because we haven't had any there. Our Homestead also was home to coyotes, dogs, mountain lions, tigers, lynxes, bobcats, foxes, raccoons, weasels, fishers, mink, pine martens, hawks, eagles, and owls — both of whom would simply enjoy a good meat lunch.

The hen we lost in the woods covered her nest and declined to be pulled into the coop. The primary reason we've had such best of luck, I think, is that we will always shut down our livestock as well as chickens farm animals night without fail. But it's hard for the predators to get direct connections once in it. Getting many big dogs around the house would aid, of course. Weasels are tiny bloodthirsty buggers.

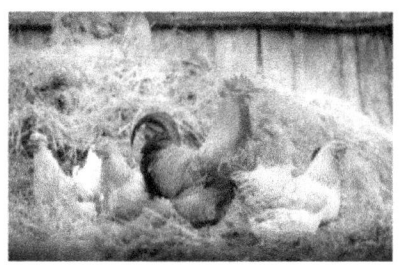

They 're very adorable, with black eyes mostly on shoe-button, alarm ears mostly on stand-up, and small little cat-like hands. They are dark with such a white belly throughout the summer but turn ermine white with such a black tip on their tail and in winter.

One weasel might squeeze the size of your thumb through a knothole, killing either of your chickens for one night. I got it completed a long time before, out on the field.

In several areas, a dog or even several loose dogs are your first dangerous creature for chicken.

They may be lovely puppies, and yet watching those loud, fluttering chickens can cause them to forget their predator and become cold.

When you stay where feral dogs play, or even pets of your neighbors, upgrading your catch with stock panels as well as electric wire is a great idea, only in case.

If raccoons tend to be prevalent in your area, I'd highly likely install a six-inch electrical wire from the bottom section of your fence as well as an appropriate string on top of the wall to avoid those sweet, furry, bloodthirsty buggers in the chicken race.

I may have killed 33 turkeys (once more on the old farm) as well as dragged them off from raccoons who crept underneath the door, smashed the window as well as chewed via the chicken wire fence. I caught five of them across the gate, killing one in the process of catching a hen from the roost—no circumstantial evidence on this level.

When hawks or owls are a concern, it's best to place netting around your outdoor run and don't allow the birds free-range. Although you do, there's just not a lot of chance to cover them. You can't carry a hawk or owl legally, so why you should.

They were doing exactly what nature had built them up to do.

Feeding the homestead flock

There is a variety of opinions about what the chickens really should be cared for. Although, Many people mainly commercial farmers and feed shop salesmen, actually recommend trying to feed your chickens with commercial feeds that match their age and only use: starting chicks, growing chicks, building broilers, egg mash, etc. Cornish Rocks are excellent processing beef.

I don't like all of the chemicals in commercial feed. Indeed, on commercial chick starter, I do launch my chicks; I didn't waste time trying to make "baby formula" as Grandma did. And as soon as they begin feathering off, I move slowly to a combined effect of decent bite feed (primarily cracked maize, millet as well as wheat); besides that, all they 're going to get drunk fresh milk. However, I've got all the kitchen scraps accessible for them as well as garden goods. My chickens scatter on all this like trees and expand to fill up my canned jars that lay all the eggs that our family would ever need.

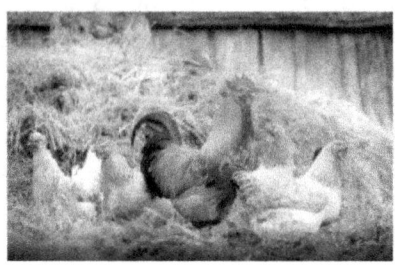

For goats and chickens, I also grow a little "special" in the garden: maize, vegetables, squash, and root crops. It's impressive how a small handful of gardeners grow year-round will slash your feed bill and improve your egg production. If I break one of our eggs open, it has an orange yolk lying squarely on the surface.

The grocery store eggs, on the other hand, are so grey because when my son David noticed that a neighbor put one in a pan, he cried out to me, "Mom! just what is wrong with the eggs?

You remember the old saying, "What are you eating? "Well, for your chickens, it's also true. Now I have seven-year-old hens, which only lay their eggs a day until they deform. Burnt up by the age of one year, industrial hens are turned into the broth. Just ask why? It's a mixture of raising a hen who lays down to death and the nutrition she needs to consume in her life.

I would like to know what kills my chickens. Try finding this out on your commercial chicken feed from the labeling.

There are things I can't pronounce here, nor even recognize what they are. Therefore the "Products" as well as "devours," etc. I feel much better to be providing real food to my chickens. When those who can't forage outside and in the winter, I still bring some carrots or vegetable crumbs from the basement with them, along with the pail of leftover food they always get every day.

They enjoy a treat of alfalfa leaves or pellets soaked in boiling water in real cold weather once they are pleasantly warm but cooled down enough just to eat.

Health Concerns:

Let me also say I have had really few sick chickens. Never. Ever. One would just die now and then. People are doing so, too. But you'll never see infected birds by feeding your flock well enough and having relatively warm, airy, dry accommodation for them. Many diseases of poultry exist only in big, commercial crowds. Which happens to a balanced bird? It is useful and vigilant. Her feathers are flat and are held close to her frame. (other than when it's a hen trying to run with roosters that will easily refuse her back multiple times through regular breeding, even when she's in molt twice a year.)

The eyes but also nostrils are free of running or crusty release. She should be feeling plump and full as you pick the chicken up. Given a health problem, a light chicken is relatively black.

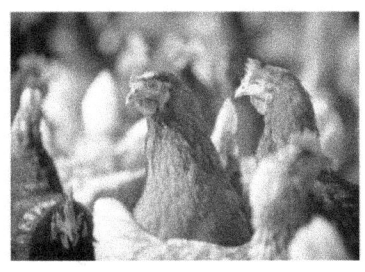

COCCIDIOSIS AND PARASITES
Parasites:
Even well looked after, flocks will sometimes pick up the external parasites, generally chicken lice or mites. By increased effectiveness and productivity of dust baths and preening, chickens would then try to keep themselves free of those. But they do need a little support sometimes. It's a good idea to capture a bird and study its skin carefully, under its wings, once in a while.

If need be, use a magnifying glass. Chicken mites are for the size of a dot made on a paper by a pencil. Lice are bigger and transparent in the color pink. Both are going to get on humans for a short period, but are not going to stay.

This is a quite frequent issue even triggered by the leg mite, the foreign parasites. You can't see these pests, so it doesn't make the ability to look for them. They make the legs raw and scaly. They cause nerve damage in severe cases, and the bird would then lose weight and then die.

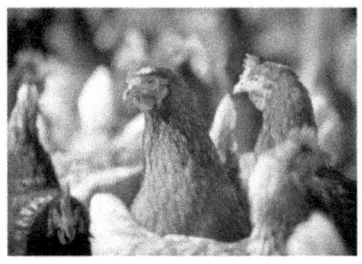

Luckily they are handled very comfortably. Simply slip the two legs into a large can of vegetable oil, a few at a time. Repeat it once a week until the legs show signs of getting better. Not only does the oil smother the mites, but it also helps relax and dissolve the scales.

COCCIDIOSIS:

Coccidiosis most commonly occurs in chicks restricted to a brooding neighborhood. It's from internal protozoa. The side effects include diarrhea, lack of strength, sitting around on those puffed up feathers as well as lacking growth. Death almost always results in untreated. Luckily, coccidiosis may easily be detected by holding the chicks under dry, clean bedding at all times. It may be treated by getting a simple sample for a fecal test for the veterinarian. Many coccidiosis situations can be treated successfully by placing the drug in the drinking water. Several veterinarians are using 2 tsp of Sulfadimethoxine. Per gallon of potable water.

Upper Respiratory problems:

So many chicken infections can turn up with illnesses of the respiratory tract. To make matters more complicated, some of these are viruses that do not have effective treatment but good care while others are bacterial and often respond to antibiotics.

The infection of the respiratory side effects includes eye as well as nostril matter, nostril discharge, sneezing, and wheezing. Many instances of upper respiratory illnesses can be attributed to two things and in the home flock: a co-op, which is continuously wet and locked in, and a dry co-op, sometimes bedded to sawdust. In all situations, it also helps to have decent ventilation.

We're not thinking about windy, just a constant cross-ventilation to hold in the fresh coop air. The warm, shuttered-in coop is often used in winter, where sure chickens are not permitted to go outside. A mixture of built-up litter and the manure-generated ammonia sets the chickens up for a severe respiratory system disease crisis. When your chickens aren't permitted out in winter, be ready to adjust bedding regularly, as well as crack open a south-facing window a bit to let in the fresh air whenever it's milder out and at least and during the daytime.

When these care tips do not have to provide immediate relief, treating the flock with an antibiotic, like Terramycin, for ten days will be a good idea. Although this won't "cure" a viral infection, it will usually take control of bacterial diseases as well as avoid a secondary infection from arising, after, or in combination with the contagious infection.

BIRD FLU:

Hey, all right. Yes, bird flu can be cached from wild birds by a flock of chickens. It is also likely they could be struck with a meteor. One virus, H5N1, causes bird flu. While present in Asia, it has not been seen in the U.S. So unless it crosses the ocean, I don't worry about that issue. Even.

If it should, I suggest isolating your flock entirely from wild birds. This includes getting them in a sealed, bird-proof coop as well as an enclosed outdoor run, which is bird-proof. The birds are likely to be safer than you will be. They don't ever go shopping, traveling, going to school, working or playing, or mixing in with the other vectors.

Chapter 13: Starting To Homestead

I'm not a farmer, nor do I have any formal agricultural training.

I am simply a man that:

• Has picked the freshest tomatoes from my grandmother's garden and ate tomato sandwiches with her for lunch.

• Learned from my grandmother that Dandelions make a great salad when you drizzle bacon grease and vinegar on top.

• Loved to shuck the corn in the brown paper bag that she brought to us for dinner.

I had never successfully grown a garden but, as a child, I had the blessings of eating from them.

And I missed that.

Fast forward to 2013...

My wife and I had spent 13 years in a townhome in the suburbs of Philadelphia, a long way and a huge cultural shift from my upbringing in rural north central Pennsylvania.

I expressed to my wife that I wanted to get back to my proverbial "roots". She, like me, grew up in the country.

So, we made a plan. We searched for a home with at least 5 acres in the Chester County area. It wasn't easy. Five acre plots are highly prized and very expensive.

We knew we would have to make sacrifices. We wrote down our goals[1] and moved forward.

Over the course of the next few weeks, we looked at numerous properties for sale. Many were too expensive or didn't offer what we were looking for.

Until...

Our Realtor called us one morning and said a new house was coming on the market. But, we needed to be forewarned that the property was still under control of the owner, but was about to go into foreclosure.

Now, my wife and I are no strangers to foreclosed properties. In our early 20's, I worked in the construction industry. The owner of the company asked my wife and I if we wanted to partner to buy and flip foreclosed houses.

We agreed.

I learned more in that one year about people than I have in 20 years. People that are going bankrupt will destroy their own houses before allowing the banks to rightfully take possession of them.

So when my Realtor told us that the home was about to go into foreclosure, I expected the worst.

We arrived at the property on a Monday morning. It was a Ranch home on 7 acres of property, mostly wooded. It was largely overgrown. There was a lot of outside work to be done, but nothing I couldn't handle.

We went inside. Upon first inspection, the home was neat and orderly. It was what we found later as we dove into the bowels of the home that we realized there would be a tremendous amount of work, but we decided it was worth the effort, so we made an offer.

Over the next six years, I would dream of starting my homestead, but for the most part, got side tracked by the ongoing upgrades I needed to make to the home we had purchased. Since moving in, we replaced the entire plumbing system (which was, at the time, a "new" plastic piping system that now had a federal class action lawsuit against it), the hot water heater, the heating and air conditioning system in total, cleaned up and upgraded the electrical system and on and on and on...

But, what I did over those six years was take a tiny step toward my homestead dreams, a couple times a year.

I didn't know where to begin the homesteading process, so I put a plan together that I knew I could manage and I started to implement it.

My homesteading started when I fertilized the wild raspberries and blackberries around my house[2]. From there, I cleaned up the front yard, ground 24 stumps and graded the soil for proper drainage.

The following year found me planting 2 apple trees.

The year after that, I found myself building 2 raised beds.

And each year after, I would add something new. Everything was going as planned. I wanted low maintenance. I wanted to be able to mow my grass, but not spend a tremendous amount of time line trimming, weeding, or mulching.

I wanted form and function.

And my planning helped me to get both.

In October of 2019, I confessed to my bride of 23 years that I was ready to go all in with homesteading.

That meant I wanted animals.

She quickly said "No."

Oof… I saw my homesteading dream starting to slip away.

Now… mind you… I may not wear the proverbial pants in my family, but I do have one thing...

I have the ability to persevere until I succeed. I always tell people, I am like water on a rock… You may think nothing is happening as water drips on a rock, but we all know that erosion is taking place and eventually the rock will disintegrate.

I planned to disintegrate my wife, metaphorically (I am a brave man stating this, as my wife is my editor and reads my books very carefully).

For months, I mentioned how much I wanted chickens. I was persistent. I continued to drip the chicken idea on her, on a weekly if not daily basis. And then, in February of 2020 I made a bold statement to my 19 year-old daughter.

"I don't care what your mother says, I am getting chickens." Notice, I didn't say it to my wife.

She simply replied, "You have to talk to mom before you do anything."

I said, "No, I don't."

She smiled at me and said, "Yes, you do." And she simply walked away.

And then it happened… COVID-19.

Lockdown.

I was glad we had started working our plan, but I decided that we needed to pick up the pace and implement faster.

At this point, no one knew what the future would hold.

My wife and I had discussed easing into homesteading with some raised beds and container gardening and that's the plan we executed on.

We had the seeds, so we started to plant.

It was early in the year and the nights were still below freezing. We decided to plant our containers first and move them out of the garage during the day and back into the garage at night to keep them from freezing.

We started our potatoes from chits[3]. Then we planted our onions, garlic (from cloves we had in our cupboard), peas, spinach, lettuce and many more items.

We were on our way.

The only guidance we had was what I remembered from my childhood and some really great articles on the internet and several YouTube channels that I followed and continue to follow.

The COVID-19 storm had literally set upon us.

Now my wife and I stood at the helm of our homesteading ship, learning how to sail it.

One day as the COVID lock downs were enforced, my wife looked at me and said, "Do you know why I didn't want you to go and buy chickens?"

I shook my head and said, "Not really, but now I wish we had."

She smiled at me. "I didn't let you buy chickens, because I already ordered them back in January for your birthday. They will arrive in a couple of weeks."

I smiled at her and gave her a hug.

Improvise, Adapt and Overcome:

We wanted to homestead but we had limited experience. We planned and planned and planned. And we learned this...

Planning is good, but you will never be able to plan for every scenario. If you want to do anything, you have to take action.

Set aside fear.

Imagine what success looks like...

Write down your goals...

And then go do it...

When COVID-19 hit, we realized that sometimes, you just need to cut the

mooring lines, set sail and weather the storms as best as you can.
And that is what we did.

Conclusion

Knowing where you're going to be is not only a physical confirmation that a new chapter is approaching, it's also a psychological one. Particularly for folks leaving the city, knowing that there is land out there that is going to be yours to work is a huge motivation as you go through the monumental process of freeing yourself from city-dependency. Furthermore, knowing if you're going to be in the mountains, in a secluded forest valley, or on a windswept plain will help you better think through the skills and tools that you might need for your new life.

If I could offer any one piece of advice, it would be to avoid getting into debt with your land purchase. Though this may not be possible with everyone's personal situation, to be able to pay for your land in cash and have it be yours and yours alone is one of the greatest freedoms, and certainly one worth saving for. If it requires you to make drastic financial changes in the meantime—selling an extra car, canceling unnecessary subscriptions, and learning to live more frugally, then you'll be developing your homesteader-mind anyway!